W9-AQX-258

Advance Praise for *The Eldercare Consultant*

"The best gift that you can give your loved one is to buy a copy of *The Eldercare Consultant*. It's a must-read for all relatives and friends struggling to cope or seeking guidance with the aging process of a loved one. The book offers a step-by-step approach to decision making, placement, and care with a very positive, kind, loving, and specific pathway. Personal stories throughout are helpful and insightful, letting readers know that they are not alone."

—*Nanci F. Scheevel, Housing Management Lead Worker, Elderly and Disabled, The Housing Authority of the County of Alameda, California*

"Author Becky Feola knows, both personally and professionally, that the role of caregiver is diverse, complex, and fraught with uncountable emotional minefields. *The Eldercare Consultant* will advise you of the pitfalls and options, ease your soul, and protect your sanity."

—*Anne L. Holmes, APR, "Boomer in Chief," National Association of Baby Boomer Women*

"*The Eldercare Consultant* is a book everyone should have on hand as aging touches their family. It comprehensively addresses not only the multifaceted needs of the elder from beginning to end but those of the caregiver as well."

—*Bridget O'Brien Swartz, Attorney, Vice President, and Senior Trust Officer, First International Bank & Trust*

"Thanks to this wonderful, comprehensive guide, the daunting and emotional task of finding and securing eldercare resources or alternative living arrangements for an aging or ill loved one just got easier. Whether the need arises from advancing age, physical challenges, or declining mental capacity, this book provides valuable insight and in-depth consideration of every aspect."

—*Joanne S. Crim, Family Caregiver*

The Eldercare Consultant

Your Guide to Making the Best Choices Possible

By Becky Feola

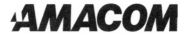

AMACOM

AMERICAN MANAGEMENT ASSOCIATION

NEW YORK * ATLANTA * BRUSSELS * CHICAGO * MEXICO CITY * SAN FRANCISCO
SHANGHAI * TOKYO * TORONTO * WASHINGTON, D.C.

Bulk discounts available. For details visit:
www.amacombooks.org/go/specialsales
Or contact special sales:
Phone: 800-250-5308
E-mail: specialsls@amanet.org
View all the AMACOM titles at: www.amacombooks.org
American Management Association: www.amanet.org

Library of Congress Cataloging-in-Publication Data

Feola, Becky.
  The eldercare consultant : your guide to making the best choices possible / by Becky Feola.
    pages cm
  Includes index.
  ISBN 978-0-8144-3631-8 (pbk.)   ISBN 978-0-8144-3632-5 (e-book)
  1. Caregivers. 2. Older people—Care. 3. Older people—Health and hygiene. I. Title.
  RA645.3.F46 2015
  613'.0438—dc23

                                                                      2015004244

About AMA
American Management Association (www.amanet.org) is a world leader in talent development, advancing the skills of individuals to drive business success. Our mission is to support the goals of individuals and organizations through a complete range of products and services, including classroom and virtual seminars, webcasts, webinars, podcasts, conferences, corporate and government solutions, business books, and research. AMA's approach to improving performance combines experiential learning—learning through doing—with opportunities for ongoing professional growth at every step of one's career journey.

Printing number
10 9 8 7 6 5 4 3 2 1

Contents

Acknowledgments

This book is dedicated to my late husband, Neil Feola Jr., who taught me about love, compassion, and unconditional commitment. You were the ultimate example of living life with dignity and passion in spite of a long and difficult battle. Not a day goes by where I don't think of you and thank you for being a part of my life. You set me on a journey of great personal growth and made me the person I am today. Shine on, my love!

I would like to express my deep gratitude to the following people who have been so important and instrumental in my life and in the process of this book.

Thank you to Judy Peters, my hospice bereavement counselor while Neil was in the last stage of his life, who is now one of my dearest friends. I'll never forget sitting on the couch with Judy toward the end, and she told me that I needed to take what I had learned during this time with Neil and to reach out to others facing similar difficulties. She said that by helping others, I would heal myself. Little did I know this conversation would lead to two elder-care businesses and a book!

Thank you to my beloved mother, Patricia Ann Bauer, whose support and insistence that I attend a fateful writers retreat in August 2012 is truly the foundation for this project of love.

Thank you to Rick Wandrych, who is my biggest cheerleader. Without your love, commitment, and never ending belief in my abilities, this book would have sat indefinitely on a dusty shelf in my mind. You believed in me and gave me the encouragement I needed to finally put pen to paper. I love you.

Thank you to Linda Sivertsen, my Book Mama, who lit the flame under me and insisted that this book needed to be written. You gave me the confidence to see what could be and exactly how I could do it. I don't believe *The Eldercare Consultant* would have made it to publishing had it not been for your support, guidance, and assistance with the proposal and with finding an agent. You are an angel!

Thank you to Jeff Herman of The Jeff Herman Agency and Bob Nirkind, Senior Acquisitions Editor for AMACOM Books. I've learned so much from both of you.

Thank you to my family—Bob, Sun, Luke, Breanna, and Colton—for your love, enthusiasm, and support! I love you all dearly.

Thank you to my mother-in-law, Barb Feola, and my late father-in-law, Neil Feola Sr.: I can't express how much your continued love and support after Neil's death has meant to me. You will always be my family.

Thank you to my friend Maryglenn Boals, who often asked those challenging questions when I was doubting myself, who kept me focused on my goal, and who made sure I knew that creating this book was important.

Thank you to the sponsors who believed there was a need for this information and supported my efforts to provide it: The National Association of Baby Boomer Women; Dr. CJ Henius, host of *Hello Dr. CJ—What's Life About*; Marketingworx PR; and Bare Essentials Marketing.

Thank you to the eldercare professionals who provide support and guidance for those in need of assistance or who are providing care for a loved one. Your input for this book was invaluable.

And finally, thank you to all the families and individuals that I have served over the years. Your personal stories are the reason this book will touch the hearts of others and will be a legacy to those we have loved and lost.

Introduction

For years, I wondered when I would know the time had come. The answer became crystal clear in the early morning hours of December 27, 2004. From the moment I walked into the kitchen and saw my husband standing at the sink, I knew my world was about to fall apart. Neil was highly agitated, glaring out the window, and talking to himself. His repetitive hand gestures and rapid eye movements had become a warning sign that he was not in a rational frame of mind. While there had been other situations where he was combative and angry, the atmosphere on this day was heavy and ominous. Though this was my husband standing before me, he was a stranger in our home.

Neil was suffering from Huntington's disease, a degenerative brain disorder. For the previous 11 years, I had watched his progressive decline. It was painful to watch his loss of mental and physical capabilities and, most recently, the development of auditory and visual hallucinations.

As I cautiously approached, he began yelling and swearing that the dogs were outside, tearing up the backyard, and that I had better do something about it. He had no awareness that our three dogs were cowering behind my legs. Within a split second, he wrapped his hand around my throat and bent my small frame backward over the granite countertop. My toes barely reached the floor as his six-foot-four frame towered over me. His eyes were wild and spit showered me with every word. Willing myself not to glance to the left, where the knives lay within inches of his reach, I was terrified of this rage and believed it was possible he could kill me. I waited for the worst. . . .

Miraculously, it ended as quickly as it began. The darkness left his eyes, his face relaxed, and he released me. Kissing me good morning, he calmly walked into the family room. Shaking uncontrollably, I dropped to the floor. There was no longer any doubt—the time had come.

I was an ordinary woman with no personal or professional training, taking care of a husband losing control of his body and mind. Within three months of our wedding, I had begun a ferocious fight for his health, dignity, and quality of life. Having vowed to love, honor, and cherish this man, it was my duty to provide and care for him until his death. Naïvely, it never occurred to me that despite our love and commitment, we would not win this battle.

On that extraordinary morning, my heart, soul, and very being broke. In a moment of clarity, I realized that I needed to do what was necessary for both of us. I was crushed when faced with the decision to have my husband committed to the hospital for observation. I was even more shaken to have the doctors tell me he would never return home and that I had 48 hours to find a group home for him. Amazingly, on the worst day of my life, I would begin a journey of hope and service for others in similar situations.

After Neil's death in April 2005, I plunged into a frenzy of activity, building two businesses that would deliver what I had so badly needed during that time: support, knowledge, and direction. Both of my companies have focused on providing families with supportive, accessible, and ethical solutions and resources for caregivers, as well as counseling, evaluations, and placement services for those seeking assisted living. Because of my firm belief that every family should know what is available to them and how to select the best care options possible, I have also regularly participated in educating people on eldercare through television and radio appearances, public seminars, as a guest lecturer for caregiver classes at local colleges, and through published articles.

When I realized that I wanted to take my expertise a step further and write a book to reach out to families providing long-term care, I reflected back on my experience with Neil. I thought about the years of visiting medical offices, attending support groups, and meeting with attorneys and financial planners. Often, we were the only two people in the waiting areas that were under the age of 65. Although there was a generational difference, our care needs were significantly similar to those seeking assistance for a beloved senior. There was no difference between me helping Neil with his daily activities and a daughter running over to her parent's home after work to help them do laundry, cook dinner, and clean up. I understood that anybody whose loved one has dementia might also experience the controlling behaviors or violence that I had. But most of all, I could see in their faces, and now in my clients' faces, that we all experience confusion and heartbreak when making difficult decisions regarding our loved ones. Every one of us is acting out of love and compassion, and though the focus of this book is on eldercare, the advice and guidance easily translate to caregivers of all ages and in all situations.

WHY THIS BOOK?

If you've bought *The Eldercare Consultant*, you're not reading it for entertainment. Something has happened or will soon be happening in your life, and you need help. I'm going to give you that help.

This book provides you with a clear, concise outline of the considerations you need to make and the steps you need to take in your new role as a caregiver. It offers practical advice; indispensable knowledge; and invaluable strategies, tools, and resources essential in guiding you through the various stages of caregiving. It aids you in making informed decisions regarding your loved one's needs and in understanding when you should seek assistance. And finally, it delivers a strong message of hope and inspiration by helping you to recognize that you are not alone in your struggles.

Caregivers such as yourself won't be the only ones who will want to have this book on hand, though. Those who come into contact with caregivers daily—be they physicians, nurses, case managers, social workers, religious or spiritual leaders, pharmacists, financial planners, or eldercare attorneys—will find it of value to their clients.

Finally, this book is not only a valuable asset to you, but it just might teach your own children how to manage your care once you require assistance!

WHAT INFORMATION WILL YOU FIND?

In order to successfully care for your loved one, you need to address a multitude of issues that you may have not previously considered. These are the concerns that catch you off guard and throw your world into chaos. By thinking ahead, considering how you would handle each situation, and preparing for those events as much as possible, you can develop a sense of control over things you can't prevent.

This book delivers clear and concise information on topics critical to understanding the full range of eldercare. The following chapter summaries provide a brief explanation of what you will find.

Chapter 1: Providing Eldercare for a Loved One

Eldercare isn't only about delivering quality care to a loved one, it's also about managing your other important relationships, such as your spouse, children, and siblings. This chapter helps you to understand how caregiving can affect these interactions and what steps you can take to nurture them. It also identifies and offers compassionate advice for the major concerns you will have in managing your loved one's care, including safety issues, functional decline, and medication management, along with how to help your senior handle major life transitions. Finally, it helps you understand your role as caregiver and that you have choices in managing your loved one's care.

Chapter 2: The Caregiver's Challenges

As a caregiver, you may find yourself overwhelmed with the many responsibilities you've taken on. Not only will you encounter changing family roles and dynamics, but you will be required to become an expert on the legalities of caregiving, management of your loved one's medical needs, handling their finances and the costs of care, identifying future needs, determining living arrangements, and helping your loved one cope with loss and death. This chapter addresses these issues and offers advice on how you can juggle your needs with caregiving, as well as how to recognize and prevent caregiver burnout.

Chapter 3: Easing Caregiver Concerns with Proactive Behavior

The key to successful caregiving is to anticipate needs and know how you will handle them rather than waiting for the crisis to happen. This chapter shows you how to identify the early warning signs, assess your loved one's requirements, and know when it's time to ask for help. It also tackles some of the more complicated issues for caregivers such as long distance caregiving, being caught between multiple generations who demand your attention, and keeping your retirement funds protected.

Chapter 4: Nurturing Your Loved One's Mind, Body, and Spirit

Care should be all encompassing. In order to safeguard your loved one's overall health, you will want to provide for his or her mental, physical, and spiritual well-being. This chapter helps you to recognize those needs and identify the steps you can take to ensure a well-balanced program of care.

Chapter 5: Considering Options for Care Needs

You don't have to go it alone. There are plenty of resources that can help. Many caregivers don't fully understand the options available to assist in providing care for their loved one. This chapter explains these possibilities, their pros and cons, and how to put that care in place, whether your desire is to provide assistance at home, hire outside help, or move a loved one to a care community.

Chapter 6: Paying for Your Loved One's Care

The biggest obstacle for many in making eldercare decisions is the cost of care. There is a risk that you may make unnecessary or poor decisions simply because you didn't understand the financial facts. This chapter helps you understand the costs and how to budget and pay for care. You may be surprised at the different methods and resources available.

Chapter 7: Having the Difficult Discussions

You've finally decided that something needs to happen, but how do you manage the emotional, and sometimes difficult, discussions with family or your loved one? This chapter offers strategies for approaching and handling conversations in order to arrive at decisions that benefit your loved one and the family as a whole.

Chapter 8: Making the Right Decision

Change is never easy, but knowing that you've educated yourself on options, talked with everyone involved in your loved one's care, and have what you need to make the best decisions possible will make it less stressful. This chapter offers advice on approaching your decision, knowing when you should compromise, and deciding who makes the final decision.

Chapter 9: Special Considerations for Care

While most people associate caregiving with the elderly and picture the normal decline that happens with aging, there are circumstances where it involves unique and often very high levels of specialized care. This chapter helps you identify if your loved one falls in a category that will require greater demands from a caregiver and whether or not you are the most capable of providing that care.

Chapter 10: Final Words of Advice
after Any Change

After all is said and done and you've put your choices into motion, there will be a period of time afterward that may make you question all your decisions. This is absolutely a normal part of the process. This chapter explains this transition period, what you should expect, and how to cope until you, your loved one, and anyone else involved in his or her care has accepted and adapted to the changes.

WHAT SPECIAL FEATURES ARE
INCLUDED IN THIS BOOK?

A unique feature of *The Eldercare Consultant* is that, throughout each chapter, there are personal stories from those who have walked in your shoes and managed different caregiving scenarios. These stories reveal how these individuals handled challenging situations and indicate the effects their decisions had on their loved one and themselves. The stories also help identify mistakes they made and what they could have done differently. Reading these first-person narratives can give you hope and validate your feelings and emotions surrounding your role as caregiver.

Another feature of this book is a Caregiver Survival Tip, featured at the end of each chapter. These tips are directly related to the chapter topic to provide you with additional ideas and useful advice.

* * * * *

When my late husband was diagnosed with Huntington's disease, I was completely unprepared for how our lives would change and what would be expected of me over the years as his caregiver. I look back now and wonder at how I ever managed his increasingly high levels of care. There was no instruction book on recognizing the signs that things were changing; no mentor to cheer me on with solid, common sense advice; and no one to hold my hand and explain that whatever I was providing for him was the best I could do. I was amazed at how little guidance was offered by his medical team—especially knowing how difficult life was going to get for both of us as his condition worsened. With *The Eldercare Consultant*, you have the support and guidance that I wish had been offered to me.

CHAPTER 1

Providing Eldercare for a Loved One

Aging—it happens to all of us. It's a natural part of life, and for anyone who has made it to his or her golden years, there will be changes and challenges to body, mind, and spirit. Bit by bit, you may notice a new wobble in your loved one's walk, an increase in those senior moments, or perhaps your older person just seems more fragile and vulnerable overall.

Providing care for a loved one will touch your life in many different ways. It might affect you personally as you care for your spouse who is recovering from a heart attack. Perhaps your best friend is a long distance caregiver for her parents living across the country. Or maybe your neighbors' elderly mother has moved in with them because she has fallen so many times, and it's not safe for her to live on her own. It would be nearly impossible to go through life and never face the aging process and some form of caregiving yourself or through someone you know.

Taking care of another person can be a tremendous responsibility, and chances are that the majority of care will fall on your shoulders. If you're lucky, you may have family members willing to help with certain issues, but it's likely that one person will be providing most of the guidance and advice to the others. Usually, there's been no special training to teach you how to manage the welfare of your loved ones before you realize it's needed, and that can be very unsettling. How do you know what you should be most concerned about? Where can you get the guidance needed to make these decisions? When will you know it's time to ask for outside help?

It's important to remember that you aren't the only one in this situation. According to research conducted by the Alzheimer's Association in 2011, there are over 43.5 million people providing care for someone over fifty years of age. But the good news is that there's a great deal of information and many resources available to assist you through the process of providing care for the aged or infirm.

IT'S NOT JUST ABOUT YOU

If you're a caregiver, not only are you significant to the person you provide care for, but you most likely also have a spouse, children, other family members, and friends who rely on you as well. Your day-to-day responsibilities and decisions affect more people than just yourself and the person for whom you are caring. They also have an impact on nearly every other person in your life. This stress can add to the normal pressures of managing your family and professional responsibilities. So who is it that may be feeling the pressure and effects of eldercare along with you?

Spouse

Providing care for another person can simply be overwhelming. It's only natural that you require a great deal of support and understanding from your significant other to manage it all. However, it's critical to remember that your significant other also has needs and that your relationship needs regular maintenance. Some suggestions for nurturing your connection are given here.

- **Talk about everything.** Couples need to be able to communicate openly and honestly. It's a must, and no subject should be off limits. Both parties need to feel that they have the right to speak about whatever is on their mind and that it will be received without judgment.

- **Listen.** It's hard to realize what your spouse is saying if you are already trying to solve the problem or form an answer in your head. Ask if your spouse is done before commenting, and it can be helpful to repeat what you heard to make sure you understood correctly.

- **Don't blame.** Blaming one another never solves the problem. Focus on what the issue is and how to solve it rather than who created it. Try to take the emotion out of the discussion and stick with the facts. Seek out ways to work as a team moving forward.

- **Don't wait too long.** Holding on to your anger, resentment, or whatever feeling is causing the stress will only delay things until a time when you can't handle it any longer and you blow up. There is always an excuse as to why you can't talk about it today, and that won't change tomorrow, next week, or next month. You need to address the issue as soon as possible and clear the air.

Children

It is not unusual for children to act out or suffer quietly when their parents are caregivers. They might be angry or anxious about what is happening within the family, sad about the changes they see in someone they love, or maybe they just feel as if they are being ignored. Here are some actions you can take to help them feel included and more secure.

- **Ask them to help.** Don't push your children aside because they are too young and you want to spare them the realities of aging. You can include them in ways that will help empower them and teach valuable life lessons and skills without exposing them to any details they are too young to understand. Explain that sharing their company, hugs, and affection is the greatest gift of all and will make anyone feel better. Also, you might prepare some topics they can talk with their loved one about. They may find that they need to initiate the conversation, but then they can sit back and simply listen to the stories. Feeling as though they are part of the process will inspire them greatly.

- **Beware of the constant crisis.** Stop and think before you react to situations. Make sure that you don't create a crisis every time something unexpected or difficult happens. Take a deep breath and ask yourself if anyone is in immediate or imminent danger. If the answer is no, then slow down, clear your head, and take time to address the situation calmly. Your children will learn from you and will develop a beneficial life skill.

- **Make time.** No matter how many different scenarios are screaming for our attention, there is always time to take a few moments, a couple of hours, or maybe even a whole day every now and then to create personal time with your children. Recognize times when your children are away from home and might be missing you, such as spending the night with friends or attending summer camp, and call them on the phone, leaving a message that tells them how much you love them and that you are proud of them. Pick a night each week and make it a mandatory family meal. Plan special dates with one child at a time, even if it's just to get an ice cream or play a game. Whatever you do, make sure that you focus on the child and create optimal quality time.

- **Invent a special nickname or habit just for them.** The comedian Carol Burnett used to sign off her variety show by tugging on her ear in honor of her grandmother to let her know how much she loved her. By giving someone a unique nickname or inventing a special action or gesture such as an ear tug, you are telling them how special they are each time you use it.

Siblings

Providing care for an aging parent or relative can bring out the best or the worst in family members. But few relationships are more emotional than those among siblings. Ideally, everyone would come together and support one another, but for various reasons, it can also

My sons were six and eight when my dad became ill. He had pancreatic cancer and we knew he wouldn't live long after the diagnosis. I was told that he would be gone within a few months, and I spent as much time as I could helping Mom care for him at their home. I was gone quite a bit, especially in the end, and slept many nights away from my family until he passed.

My husband and I tried to protect our kids by not involving them in the day-to-day stuff regarding his care and declining health. Whenever we visited Dad or he came to our house, we tried to behave as though everything was OK, but they would always act out and be distant to him. He would try to hug them and they'd push him away. They'd also demand attention from us at inappropriate times. My youngest became very argumentative at school.

I knew that they were feeling left out and angry. Since Dad died, they are still very clingy and demanding and keep asking if Grandma's going to get sick too, and am I going to live with her then. I realize now that I should have taken a different approach with them. They didn't understand and felt abandoned by me. –*Toni* end with strained relationships or conflicts. Why? The demands of caring for an aging loved one will invariably give rise to old family dynamics and patterns. Adult children may find themselves replaying old hurts and resentments and reopening those wounds, making it difficult to work together. There may be a sibling who is in denial over the condition of the parent and who refuses to be involved because he or she doesn't want to face the truth. Another sibling may feel responsible for the majority of or all the caregiving duties due to close geographical proximity or fewer outside responsibilities than the others. Whatever the case, there are ways in which families can come together in the best interests of all concerned.

- **Ask for open and honest communication.** Let everyone know that their feelings and opinions matter.

- **Keep everyone informed of a loved one's condition.** Use e-mail and group settings to make it easy to send one e-mail with all the information rather than to make time-consuming personal calls to each family member.

- **Have realistic expectations.** People have different skills and abilities. One person may be quite good at hands-on care such as showering and dressing a loved one, while another may balk at such intimate assistance but will excel at managing money. Accept them for who they are and what they can provide.

- **Respect differences of opinions.** You may not always carry out another's wishes, but you can show respect and acknowledge each other's feelings. Find ways to compromise whenever possible. Remember, there is usually more than one way to do something.

- **Utilize other professional services.** If discussions are too heated, find a mediator such as a social worker, religious leader, or counselor to facilitate family meetings. If siblings are unable to help with care, find outside agencies to come in and provide respite, help with meals, or offer companion services. There are many resources available if you are willing to move beyond the idea that you should only rely on family support.

Friends

Friendships are often a lifeline for a caregiver. It's not uncommon for a friend to provide more comfort and support than family members. But caregiving can also take a toll on these bonds, and it takes effort from both sides to make it work. You can ensure your friendships will last while your focus increases on an aging loved one by taking certain steps.

- **Share openly and honestly.** While you don't want to dominate every conversation with the details of providing care, do let your friends know that your time is limited because of care-related appointments or that you're feeling run down and need to nap instead of having coffee. If you are straightforward about how you're feeling or what challenges you have right now, your friends will understand.

- **Be a good friend back.** Remember that just because you are struggling with your own situation, your friends still have lives they are living as well. Make sure you ask how they are, what their kids have been up to, or if anything new happened in their lives. Show an interest in them and then listen!

- **Ask for specific help.** Your friends want to be there for you, but it can be extremely frustrating if you won't tell them what they can do. Many have no clear idea of what would be helpful. If you need someone to spend an hour with your mother so you can take a bubble bath, say so. Maybe you'd like for someone to fix a meal or pick up a meal from a restaurant to give you a break from cooking and cleaning, so ask for that. The key is to be specific, and you may find that you get exactly what you want or need.

- **Identify friends from acquaintances.** It can be heartbreaking when you realize that someone you thought was a friend is not acting like one, especially when you are in need. It can be extremely helpful to take account of your relationships and identify whom you believe you can truly turn to in a time of need. Don't waste precious time and energy investing in a person who doesn't fall into that category, and you will free up more time for those who do.

Professional Relationships

Maintaining your work responsibilities and relationships can be one of the biggest challenges while providing care. You can take the following steps to care for your loved one without jeopardizing your career.

- **Understand your rights at work.** Your first step in maintaining your professional relationship is to learn what your rights and protections are at work with regard to caring for parents or other loved ones. The Federal Family and Medical Leave Act of 1993 (FMLA) allows employees to take 12 weeks unpaid, job protected leave for the purpose of providing care for a spouse, parent, or child with a serious health condition.

- **Inform your employer of your needs.** Contact your supervisor or the human resources department at your place of work and let them know about your situation. Discuss any possible changes to work hours, work environment, or time off you may need. It may be possible that you can work more flexible hours or telecommute in lieu of taking leave.

- **Always be professional.** While our employer and fellow employees may be kind, supportive, and understanding of your situation, you must remember to always behave as a professional during business hours. Don't use your employer's time to make personal phone calls or waste another employee's time by sharing your troubles during working hours. Focus on continuing to perform your duties at your highest level, even though you may be feeling emotional. The bottom line is that you need to maintain and honor your business relationships to protect your income and future.

Being a caregiver for a loved one is a rewarding experience. However, being thoughtful about your other relationships can also promote a sense of normalcy and peace for you, your family, and everyone else included in your daily life.

YOUR BIGGEST CONCERNS REGARDING ELDERCARE

Decisions about providing care for another individual are not easy. There are many worries that can overwhelm and confuse those in charge of managing that care. The good news is that you can and should prioritize these concerns. You don't need to spend a great deal of effort and thought on every need or desire your loved one may have. Give yourself some breathing room. Start with the major areas you should be focusing on and then, when you are confident these are being managed appropriately, you can begin concentrating on the smaller needs.

Safety

Ask those who are providing care for an elderly person what they most worry about, and certain images will likely come to mind: their loved one falling with no help close by; becoming confused while driving and turning in front of oncoming traffic; or, one of the most

Our family is very small. There are only my parents who are in their eighties and my husband, Carl, and me. Carl's retired, but I still work for a large marketing firm and have another eight years until my retirement. Carl goes over to their home every day and helps with maintaining their yard or household repairs and makes sure they get to and from any appointments they have. I go over at least four or five times during the week and every day on the weekend. We were raised to honor and respect our parents, and it is our responsibility to care for them.

Over the past year, I realize that Carl and I have grown apart in some areas. We are more like friends than husband and wife. I think we don't spend enough time with each other and nurturing our relationship. We've been to a few counseling sessions and have learned that we can't let my parents' declining health and needs become the only focus in our life together. We need to carve out time to concentrate on each other. Although our desire to provide care for my parents is commendable, we realize that both of us don't need to visit every day, and we can put some services in place such hiring a yard and housecleaning service. Another change is that I'm dedicating one day only to cooking and freezing all their meals for a week. Since I don't have to cook every evening and the weekends for them, Carl and I can enjoy eating together again. Also, we purchased an emergency alert system for them that will allow us to relax and take some mini vacations away from home knowing that they can get help if needed.

After seeing how well these changes were working for everyone, I decided to talk with the human resources department about reducing the number of hours I work each week. They were fine with me cutting back to three days a week in the office and telecommuting from home the other two. This will allow even more flexibility and freedom for both Carl and me.

> Overall, Carl and I are reconnecting with each other, and we're now reaching out to spend time with friends that we've lost touch with. Caring for my parents is a wonderful experience, but I'm so happy we've taken steps to make sure our lives are balanced and that we are caring for our marriage and ourselves as well. *–Fran*

dangerous, growing forgetful and taking a medication in the morning and then again later, resulting in an overdose. The best factor for determining what one should worry most about is whether it pertains to the safety or essential health and well-being of an individual. This takes priority over those that deal with personal preferences or desires. Some of the major issues that should be watched for and addressed in a timely manner include the following items.

- **Home environment.** For most, safety begins at home. Conduct a thorough inspection of the living environment and assess any hazards that might cause a fall or injury, such as throw rugs and out of place furniture. Can there be a fire risk because of piles of magazines or newspapers? Are the air conditioning and heating units working properly? Do the windows and doors lock and unlock easily? Is the lighting adequate inside and out? If you aren't sure you are catching all the potential hazards, there are home safety assessment tools available online, or you can hire someone to conduct the assessment in person and make recommendations to make the property safe.

- **Abuse or neglect.** Every person has the basic human right to be free and safe from all forms of abuse or neglect. *Physical abuse* results in pain, injury, or impairment. Symptoms will include bruising, swelling, cuts or scratches, or even broken bones. *Emotional abuse* causes emotional pain or distress. It is caused by intimidation through yelling and threats, humiliation or ridicule, ignoring the person, isolation, and other forms of menacing behaviors. *Sexual abuse* involves physical sexual acts, but may also include exposing a person to pornographic material.

- **Neglect or abandonment.** This may or may not be intentional, but neglect or abandonment is a failure to support the physical, emotional, and social needs of the person in your care. *Neglect* is usually the result of caregivers feeling overwhelmed or overloaded and might be identified as not providing enough food, withholding medications, physically restraining a person, or confining a person in his or her room or home with no stimulation. *Abandonment* is when a person is completely deserted with no support.

- **Financial exploitation.** This involves unauthorized use of a person's funds or property. It can include the misuse of a person's checks, credit cards, cash, or household goods. Forging a person's signature or committing identity theft is also classified as exploitation.

Functional Decline

Functional decline is the loss of the ability to do certain things. For a loved one who is aging or already elderly, it will become more prominent over time. The following are some of the signs of functional decline.

- **Physical symptoms.** This includes changes to or loss of vision, hearing problems, balance issues or falls, decreased mobility, trouble sleeping or eating, incontinence or lack of hygiene, and skin problems, including pressure sores.

- **Mental or emotional symptoms.** This includes changes in personality, memory loss, depression, and behavioral problems.

Every human being experiences some functional decline with age. However, there are some things you can do to ensure that you and your loved ones remain as healthy and independent as possible.

- **Get enough sleep.** Six to nine hours each night should be the goal.

- **Watch your diet.** Make sure your meals are full of healthy and nutritious foods. Avoid sugar and processed foods.

- **Stay hydrated.** This is especially critical for our elderly loved ones who can develop conditions such as urinary tract infections that can land them in the hospital.

- **Exercise.** Keeping our bodies moving is necessary to maintain muscle mass and flexibility and to reduce falls. As they say, "A body in motion tends to stay in motion."

- **Keep your brain healthy.** All of the above will assist in keeping your brain healthy but also make sure your loved one is receiving as much social stimulation as possible and participating in activities such as reading; watching television programs that require thought, like game shows where the viewer can answer questions or play along with contestants; and engaging in hobbies or taking courses on subjects that are of interest. One of the most important things you can do to keep your brain healthy is to keep stress under control. Find ways to manage stress through meditation, deep breathing, or visualization.

Falls

Falling can happen at any age, but it can be particularly serious for the elderly, who are at higher risk for serious complications from brittle bones or other medical conditions. A younger person may recover quickly, but a fall for an older person may result in an emergency trip to the hospital. In some cases, it can lead to a loss of mobility and independence, traumatic brain injury, or possibly death. The good news is that there are easy ways to help prevent falls from happening.

- **Keep your environment clear.** A cluttered living space will invite accidents. Make sure throw rugs are tossed out, remove unnecessary furniture such as low-lying coffee tables or stools, secure loose cords or wires, and pick up shoes or clothing strewn about on the floor. Anything you can remove from pathways will help reduce the risk of falling.

- **Build muscle strength.** Exercise will develop muscle strength and thereby increase a loved one's balance and ability to recover at the beginning of a fall.

- **Check your medications and supplements.** Many medications such as sedatives or antidepressants may cause fatigue, dizziness, or other side effects that might make your loved one more susceptible to falling. Make a list of all medications and supplements, take it to your doctor or your pharmacist, and ask if they might increase your loved one's risk of falling. If the answer is yes, then discuss what might be eliminated to help promote safety.

- **Get a checkup.** Many health issues can contribute to your loved one being unsteady on his or her feet—like eye or ear problems. Take your loved one to visit your doctor or specialists to ensure there aren't any conditions that might need treatment.

Medication Management

It's been estimated that over 50 percent of seniors will mismanage their medications and that over 10 percent of all hospital admissions are a direct result of that mismanagement. This is one of the most serious concerns for seniors and their families. Not taking medications properly can result in hospitalization or worse—death. There are many reasons why people may not take their meds properly. Here are some of the more common excuses and suggestions on how to resolve them.

- **I forgot to take my pills.** While it can be true that they simply forgot, neglecting to take pills may also be caused by memory issues or the side effects of medications. The family may want to consider pill organizers, services that provide reminder phone calls, or watch alarms that sound when it's time to take their medications.

- **I can't read the prescription labels.** If they can't read the label to know how much to take or what pills they are taking, seniors may simply choose not to take their medications at all. The solution is quite easy. Ask the pharmacist to use large print on the labels. Make sure loved ones have a magnifying glass nearby to help read smaller print. Or, once again, have a family member fill up a pill organizer.

- **I can't afford the medication.** Financial difficulty leads many seniors to either stop taking their medications, purchase larger pills and split them, or take them at irregular intervals to make them last longer. This can be disastrous. It can lead to health complications, overdoses, or even death. For lower income families, there can be relief by requesting generic brand drugs, asking your pharmacist if they offer any discount drug programs, and researching prescription assistance programs through online organizations such as BenefitsCheckup.org.

Dementia

Dementia is not a disease in itself. It's a collection of symptoms caused by a number of disorders that affect the brain. In general, it's a decline in mental function that is severe enough to interfere with daily life. Dementia can cause many issues for your loved one and family members. The symptoms can include the following:

- becoming lost in familiar places or wandering away from home
- being unable to follow directions
- losing orientation about times, places, and people
- asking the same questions or making the same statements over and over
- lacking the ability to make sound judgments, especially about money
- losing the ability to communicate
- neglecting personal hygiene, nutrition, and safety

These symptoms can place tremendous stress on caregivers, especially if they are accompanied by severe changes in behavior.

The symptoms of dementia vary greatly, but a diagnosis of dementia requires that two of the following core mental functions must be significantly impaired:

- memory
- communication and language
- ability to focus and pay attention
- reasoning and judgment
- visual perception

It is important to remember that many people may develop memory issues that are classified as dementia. Medications, infections, and acute illness are some of the causes of memory loss that could possibly be reversed with treatment.

To date, dementia is not curable, but there are great strides being made in the efforts to find cures or treatments such as gene therapy, stem cell therapy, and dementia vaccines. There is also the positive news that some of the symptoms may be treatable, at least for a period of time, to provide relief to both the patient and the caregivers.

If you suspect that your loved one has dementia, it is critical to schedule a doctor's visit as soon as possible for a thorough evaluation. Here are some things to help prepare for the appointment.

- Make a list of mental and physical complaints and any unusual behaviors.

- Make a list of all medications and supplements, including both prescription and over-the-counter.

- Consider scheduling an appointment with the doctor for yourself to provide essential information and address your concerns before meeting together with your loved one. This will allow you to provide helpful information without causing discomfort, embarrassment, or fear for your loved one.

Finally, if there is a diagnosis of dementia, surround yourself with as much support as possible. Seek out support groups, educate yourself about the condition causing the dementia, and when things get really difficult, remember that it's OK to love the person you're caring for, but you don't have to love the disease.

Isolation

Mental and social stimulation are tremendously important to a person's overall well-being. When people are isolated, they will decline physically and mentally much faster than if they are in an environment that will provide much-needed interaction. Isolation can cause the following:

- aches and pains, headaches, illness, or other medical conditions

- anxiety, panic attacks, depression, or paranoia

- tiredness

- lack of motivation

- difficulty sleeping

- weight gain or loss

- loss of appetite

- substance abuse

- low self-esteem, hopelessness, and thoughts of suicide

If you're worried about your loved one feeling isolated, there are things you can do to help.

- **Help them to connect or reconnect with family and friends.** Reach out to let family and friends know your loved one wants a relationship and would love to see them in person, talk on the phone, read letters and cards, or even use the computer to stay in touch.

- **Yes, use the computer.** While many seniors feel that Skyping and social media are not proper ways to interact with family and friends, it is more likely that they are uncomfortable using a computer. Invest some time helping them learn how and you may have a hard time getting them off at the end of the day! As their confidence grows, not only will they be able to communicate with others, but they may even learn how to play games, use brain fitness programs, and engage in other positive activities that will take their mind off of their loneliness or depression.

- **Suggest a pet if they don't have one.** Pets make excellent companions and provide a sense of purpose.

- **Help them get out and about.** Investigate means of transportation so they can get out on their own, if possible. Being able to run errands, going out to eat, or seeing a movie will give them more independence and help with self-esteem and happiness.

Depression

Significant life events or the changes in your loved one's body can cause depression. The death of a spouse and friends, medical problems, a reduced sense of purpose, or the loss of independence can all lead to moodiness, sadness, or worse. Depression is common in older adults or those who are debilitated, but it doesn't have to be a part of your loved one's life. Depression can be easily treated with medication, therapy, or a change in lifestyle. The key is to recognize it and seek help. Here are some of the clues that a person is depressed:

- feelings of hopelessness or helplessness

- anxiety and excessive worries

- irritability

- loss of interest in things that use to give pleasure

- memory problems

- lack of motivation or energy

- neglect of personal care, such as showering or eating

- unexplained aches and pains

- thoughts of suicide or death

Depression is a serious medical condition and needs to be addressed as soon as possible. In addition to seeking treatment, there are some things you can do to help your loved ones.

- Accompany them to doctor appointments and offer support.

- Listen to what they say and don't judge; give them feedback based on reality and hope.

- Encourage them to interact with others and to take care of themselves.

- Make sure they are taking their medications.

MANAGING LIFE TRANSITIONS

Life is simply a series of transitions. From the time we're small children stepping into school for the first time and then graduating from college, getting married, and having children, it's expected that we will learn, grow, and adjust. But certain changes in life are overwhelming to us all and more so for the elderly, who may have health problems, suffer from memory loss, be more fragile because of age, or be set in their ways and simply stubborn. It's possible that they'll need a little more support and assistance to get through these moments than a younger person will in order to make it less stressful.

Retirement

One of the first major transitions an older person will have to navigate is leaving the workforce. For many people, their profession is their entire identity. *"I've been a doctor for 40 years. What will I do with myself if I quit working?"* Retirement can have a different effect on each person, but for most it will mean reduced income, changing roles or relationships, and having nowhere to go and nothing to do. While some look forward to quitting work and spending more time on hobbies, family, and self, for others it may mean hours of feeling bored and unproductive.

Loss of income is often the culprit for much of the anxiety retirement causes. Without money, seniors may not be able to afford to take the trips they dreamed of, may have to downsize because their home is now too big and too expensive, and may no longer have enough money coming in to pay for rent, food, and medications. Budgeting beforehand and preparing for retirement would be ideal, but it's equally important afterward. You may have to sit down with your loved ones and insist on going over the finances together in order to help them find ways to manage.

Along with the loss of income also comes the loss of the relationships with the coworkers they interacted with daily. This can be as depressing as losing a good friend. In fact, they may have just lost all their friends, especially if they were a workaholic. They've also lost their ability to control and manage others, which is why you often hear of the cliché where the husband is now micro managing his wife's daily chores and activities.

Finding interests and activities to replace the daily routine of work is necessary to maintain mental and emotional health. If your loved one is really struggling with retirement, perhaps volunteering with charitable organizations or groups, joining a club, or taking classes on engaging subjects will help ease the transition.

Relocation

By the age of retirement, many people find themselves living in a house much larger than they need or more expensive than they can now afford. Children have grown and don't visit as often as was planned; two people don't need four bedrooms and three baths or the yard with the swimming pool, basketball hoop, and playhouse. These big homes often require too much work and money to maintain. Perhaps your loved one would simply like to focus on other things. Unfortunately, declining health may dictate the need for new living arrangements. No matter what the driving force is, the thought of downsizing, selling a home, and moving can be very unsettling. It can be so overwhelming that some people will simply refuse to even think about it and remain in a situation that isn't in their best interest. Depending on the reason for the move, you can assist them by listening to their thoughts and feelings on the matter and then providing resources to assist them.

Maybe a little counseling is needed, or the assistance of agencies that specialize in downsizing and that can help them sort through their possessions, decide what to do with them, and then make the arrangements so that the process is not so overwhelming. Doing your homework and having the support identified and available will help make an overwhelming project much more bearable.

Taking the Car Keys Away

At some point in time, it will be inevitable. It will no longer be safe for your loved one to drive. This may be the most traumatic transition he or she faces. It means a loss of independence and, for many, the end of the road. No pun intended. While giving up the keys may mean more of an inconvenience to getting around, it doesn't mean that your loved one will become a prisoner. There are plenty of options to help her maintain that independence if she is willing to meet you halfway.

- **Be realistic and prepared to have a series of discussions.** It is highly unlikely one discussion will resolve the issue. Don't be surprised if emotions run high and your loved one becomes very angry and refuses to talk further. Avoid coming on too strong in the beginning. Ask some questions that will force her to reflect on her driving skills, such as *"Are you aware that you drive with the passenger side in the bike lane?"* or *"What do you think about the fact that you've been in two fender benders this month?"* She is probably already aware of the difficulties, and this will allow her to acknowledge her own concerns. If she becomes defensive, be willing to back off, but firmly set the expectation that there will be another conversation when she has calmed down.

- **Listen and reflect.** Give her time to talk about her feelings and fears. You may find her reminiscing about the past and giving you reasons why she can't give up driving. Talking through her driving life may make it easier to reach the conclusion that it may be time to give it up. Ask why she thinks it might be time to stop, and then offer your reasons, such as the amount of money she will save on gas, insurance, parking, and perhaps car payments. Remind her that there are plenty of ways to get around without owning a car. Be prepared to tell her exactly what those options are—such as using Dial-a-Ride, calling a cab, or utilizing the senior center's bus—and how much they may cost. Reassure her that you will help until she is comfortable making arrangements on her own.

- **Seek out a second or third opinion.** Sometimes our opinions don't carry much weight. It might be necessary to bring in an expert to convince your loved one it is time. Our seniors respect certain authority figures such as their doctors, religious leaders, or police officers. Bring the subject up with someone you know your loved one respects and ask that person for help. That may be all it takes: to have someone else whom she trusts and listens to tell her that she shouldn't be driving. Or you can insist on a driving test and then let that be the deciding factor, at least for the time being.

- **Disable the car.** If all else fails and you believe that your loved one is highly likely to hurt herself or another, then you may need to take extreme measures such as disabling the car. If the car won't run, then she can't drive.

Death and Dying

Perhaps the most difficult transition to cope with is when seniors begin losing their friends and are facing their own mortality. Coping with death can be difficult for anyone, but when compounded with issues such as declining health and memory loss, it can be an even

During the past year, my brother and I had a discussion and found out that we were both terrified to be in a car with Mom when she was driving. She'd had a stroke that affected her right eye, and she now had trouble discerning where she was on that side, so she tended to drive to the far right. She also drove too fast. So when she would try and pass other cars, we felt like we were going to clip them and everyone would end up in the ditch.

Several conversations regarding giving up the keys had gone very badly, and there were times she wouldn't talk to us. Finally, a friend suggested we tell her that if she would go to the DMV, take their test and pass it, we would stop asking her to give up her car. She was so confident that we were wrong, she immediately agreed.

Needless to say, she did not pass the test. She was still angry that she failed, but she couldn't blame us and now the state had taken her license away and it's their fault, not ours. –*Callie*

greater struggle. While there is no right way to help someone deal with grief, there are some things you can do.

- **Acknowledge the loss.** Tell him you understand it must be difficult, and ask him to share stories with you about the person who has died.

- **Listen attentively.** Don't be too eager to share your feelings or to make comments. He may need to tell the same story over and over until he comes to terms with the death. If he doesn't want to talk, be willing to sit quietly with him if he would like.

- **Be understanding.** Not everyone grieves in the same manner. Don't tell him how he should handle it. Be respectful of the process, but let him know that you are there for support.

Providing care for a loved one is often a long, complicated journey. You can drive yourself crazy thinking about every concern or issue that might arise. My advice is to remember that not every concern is critical or needs to be addressed as a crisis. One fire at a time . . . slow down, breathe deep, and think carefully about where you need or want to spend your energy and time. You'll want to acknowledge the situation in its entirety, but you'll also find it much easier to handle if you prioritize regularly—maybe even daily.

RECOGNIZING YOUR ROLE AS A FAMILY CAREGIVER

"I'm not a caregiver. He's my husband, and it's my job to take care of him." I can't tell you how many times I've heard a similar version of this statement. Family members in particular tend to view the role of caregiver more along the lines of an extended version of their relationship with the person receiving care or providing care. Why is it so important to identify yourself as a family caregiver? Mostly because if you don't call yourself a caregiver, you will never reach out for support, resources, or solutions that might be available to you. You, and perhaps others, tend to see it as a role that requires you to do it all. And that's not true at all!

You might think to yourself that it doesn't really matter what you're called, but it does. Sometimes the role of caregiver sneaks up on you. Over time, you begin to assume more and more responsibilities while taking care of yourself and others that you don't even realize you are a caregiver. You're just doing it, and by the time you realize it, you're overwhelmed, exhausted, and sometimes desperate. Caregiving can cause stress, emotional and physical problems, financial struggles, and much more, so being able to identify yourself as a caregiver may prompt you to claim your right to also care for yourself. This will then enable you to provide better care for your loved one.

Did you know the following facts?

- Family caregivers who live with their loved one spend an average of 39.3 hours per week providing care.

- Caregivers show higher levels of depression, as well as exhibiting other mental health problems such as anxiety, stress, frustration, and feelings of loneliness or isolation.

- They are also more susceptible to substance abuse or dependence, smoking, and consuming more saturated fat.

- Caregivers suffer from more physical ailments such as headaches, pain/aching, diabetes, arthritis, cancer, obesity, slower wound healing, high blood pressure, higher levels of cholesterol, and an increased risk of heart disease.

- They report lower levels of self-care such as engaging in preventive health behaviors, visiting their own doctors, exercising, and eating healthy.

- Approximately 60 percent of caregivers die before their care receivers.

The good news is that being a family caregiver also has a positive side. Caregivers often report positive feelings of being useful, having a sense of self-worth, a greater confidence in their abilities, and an increased family closeness. Some even say that they have gone through spiritual growth that may not have happened otherwise. Lastly, caregiving often requires complex thought that can ward off cognitive decline.

How Do You Know If You Are a Caregiver?

A few simple questions may give you clear insight on whether or not you should accept the title of "caregiver."

- Who does your loved one depend on the most?

I have been caring for my widowed mother for several years. Although she is still very sharp mentally, she is physically fragile. I go to her house each morning and help her shower and dress for the day because she's had several falls first thing after she wakes up. Then I cook her breakfast and lunch before I head off for work. Also, I stop by on my way home from work and either cook dinner or we go out to eat. Although she takes great pride in tidying up her home during the day, I still have to do a deeper cleaning on the weekends and wash her laundry. And I miss a lot of work taking her to various appointments. Thank God, I'm a real estate agent and can choose my own hours.

Mom recently asked me if we could go to a seminar on benefits for the surviving spouses of veterans. My dad fought in the Korean War, and she was wondering if there was any money she might be entitled to. Yes, there is. It's called the Aid and Attendance Benefit and it would pay for caregivers to come in to the home to help her. Interestingly, the caregivers can be a family member other than a spouse, a friend or they can be professional providers. More importantly, I realized that I am considered her caregiver because I'm providing this help. My mom can actually pay me with this benefit and I don't have to suffer from missing out on clients if I want to continue helping her myself. This is great because I truly enjoy the time I have left with my mom and taking care of her.

Funny, I never thought of myself as her caregiver. I'm just her daughter doing what a daughter should do. It's nice to realize how others see my role and that there's help for me financially to make it happen. –*Anne*

- Who would your loved one call in the case of an emergency?
- Who handles medications and doctor's appointments?

Caregiving is hard work. Take vacations, also known as respite, just like you would for any other job.

Accept help. When people offer, be specific, let them know what you need, and then let them do it.

Learn as much as you can about your loved one's condition. Knowledge is power, especially when dealing with medical personnel and insurance companies.

Trust your instincts. You know your loved one better than anyone.

- Who knows the most about your loved one's condition and care needs?

- Who does the hard, intimate work, such as helping with showers and toileting?

Owning your role as caregiver will allow you to acknowledge how much you do for your loved one. It will give you a sense of responsibility to the person you are caring for and to yourself, giving you permission to take care of yourself so you can continue to take care of your loved one.

You Have Choices in Managing Care

You have now identified the main concerns regarding aging and eldercare. You've also realized and acknowledged that you are a caregiver. Right about this time, you may be scared to death over what this means. Don't be. There are many choices and resources available for every type and every level of need. Taking a realistic look at what your loved one needs, what you are truly capable of providing, and who to turn to for help when it becomes more than you can deliver will be the first steps in making sure that there is as high of a quality of life for all involved. Whether you choose to provide care through the family, bring on professional caregivers, or move your loved one to a care community, you will do it knowing that you've educated yourself and are making informed decisions.

CHAPTER 2

The Caregiver's Challenges

Being a caregiver can be one of the most rewarding experiences you will ever have. Many consider having tended to a vulnerable loved one among their greatest accomplishments. However, many caregivers don't take into consideration the level of physical, emotional, or financial commitment that role may require. Most have never had to provide care for an aging loved one before and have no experience or knowledge of how they should proceed and what trials they will face.

A major factor affecting how challenging the duty of care will be is whether or not you saw it coming. It's definitely easier if, over time, you observed your love one's slowly increasing need for assistance. That lead time allows you to start discussing your role in your loved one's care with him or her, learning what options are available, putting resources in place, and asking others for help. It's more likely that your introduction to the role of caregiver will be an unexpected event that alerts you to the fact your loved one needs assistance, such as a holiday visit where you notice that your parents can no longer maintain their home or should not be driving. If there's been an emergency, there may be limited or no choices at all.

The best mantra you can have when watching over an aging loved one is "Hope for the best, but prepare for the worst." Both you and your loved one will benefit if you become a strong advocate for yourself as well as for your senior. Recognizing what challenges you may face, determining priorities, investigating resources, and forming a plan are important steps to successful caregiving. Being proactive in planning and decision making, rather than reactive to an emergency, can make all the difference. Let's examine some of the major concerns you may face when accepting the role as caregiver.

CHANGING FAMILY DYNAMICS

The roles and expectations for family members become muddled or change altogether when a loved one needs to rely on others for assistance. Sometimes the changes are minor. Perhaps your mother can no longer drive, but she is still able to manage other activities of daily life such as cooking, cleaning, and handling her finances without help. As of now, she only needs you to provide transportation. In this instance, your roles change very little. However, as she continues to age, begins to struggle more with these activities, and requires additional assistance, the roles start to shift, sometimes dramatically. It's not only the parent/child relationship that undergoes transformation; other family members can be affected as well.

When Roles Reverse Between Parent and Child

Possibly the most difficult change in the family dynamic is when a parent needs to depend on a child to provide care. Throughout our childhood, our parents are the decision makers and the ones we turn to for support and comfort. It's hard when the tables turn and they require our assistance, especially if they are resistant to the change or don't agree with our choices.

Unless your loved one has severe cognitive decline, has been declared incompetent, or has legally given you full control over her affairs and well-being, it can be helpful to understand that you are not there to "parent." Your responsibility is to help her deal with the changes that come with aging, to acknowledge that help is needed, and to encourage her to accept whatever that help may be.

If you develop an attitude that you are "in charge" now and that your parents will do what you tell them, you are most certainly going to find your relationship altered and problematic. You can avoid this trap and successfully provide guidance, support, and care without damaging your relationship by taking certain steps.

- **Focus on communication.** Open and honest communication, where both parties can express their feelings and concerns, will protect against the caregiver's actions becoming too parental.

- **Recognize limitations and respect boundaries.** Remember that not every parent and child has the type of relationship where either would be comfortable with some aspects of caregiving, like assistance with showering or toileting.

- **Assess the situation together.** Discuss the signs that help is needed and what help might be available. Be aware that there may be more than one way to provide care, and remember that your loved one has a say in how it's accomplished.

- **Foster your loved one's independence.** Resist the temptation to take over and do everything for your loved one. If it's safe, allow her to try, even if she is slightly struggling.

Recognizing Siblings and Other Family Members as Caregivers

Often, one family member is designated as caregiver, and the rest of the family is happy to defer to that person. There can be times where more than one person wishes to have a say or participate in the caregiving, though. This can result in hurt feelings or conflict if all parties

I became my 92-year-old father's caregiver two years ago after he had a stroke and could no longer live on his own. He fully recovered, but my wife and I realized he was physically too fragile to manage his home. We decided he would move in with us.

Shortly after, we realized that he was also incontinent and unable to fully clean up after an accident. I started helping him with toileting and showering. He quickly became very confrontational. We tried to monitor him, but every time we asked if he needed to go to the bathroom, he would snap at us. "Don't treat me like a child." I think it was humiliating for him to have me wiping him and seeing him naked.

Three months after moving in, I decided that something needed to change. This situation was just too emotional and embarrassing. I felt like my whole relationship with Dad was failing.

I contacted an in-home care agency that sent out a beautiful young woman to talk with Dad about the new "adult brief" available and possibly having an aide help him shower. She was very knowledgeable in how to talk with him about wearing protection in a way that didn't demean him, and he agreed immediately. It helped that she was so pretty; he was completely charmed. During the discussion, she also learned that he was fine with anyone helping him shower other than a family member. Finally, she stressed to him that as long as he managed his toileting, nobody in the family would have to help him, but if he wasn't successful, my wife or I would still have to help.

That was all it took and Dad became intent on not having any accidents. I've stopped checking on him and he's doing fine. I understand how he must have felt. No son should see his father naked and embarrassed under those circumstances. Thankfully, our relationship is back to normal. —*Owen*

aren't considered. Relationships can be damaged or ended over the choices surrounding the care of a mutual loved one. For instance, if your mother and her sister are extremely close and you don't consult with the aunt over major changes, or if you don't include your siblings in any decisions and refuse to accept their suggestions, resentment and conflict can develop. You can ensure that other family members feel included and preserve your relationship with them by taking the following steps.

- **Designate caregiving roles.** If there is more than one person who wants to provide support, determine each person's role and responsibilities. If one child is a CPA and wants to handle the finances, assign that responsibility to that person. If another family member wants to wash and style her hair each week, welcome the offer of assistance. Or, if a relative, who lives out of state, can't participate in the day-to-day care but wants to be included, that person could be asked to handle research on issues like finding a more affordable prescription program or the cost of repairs to the home.

- **Communicate effectively.** If you are the primary caregiver, but there are others who want to be kept abreast of the situation, don't withhold information because you're too busy and stressed. You don't have to take the time to e-mail or call each person separately. Set up groups in your e-mail so you can notify people all at once and ask for help in calling those who don't use e-mail. Also consider using social media, like creating a private Facebook page just for family and friends, to stay updated and connected.

- **Seek mediation, if necessary.** If you recognize that there is too much conflict or negative emotion to effectively work together with others, seek professional help. Find a family counselor or mediator and ask for that professional's guidance or to make the final decisions.

In an ideal situation, all family members will communicate openly, honestly, and respectfully. They will work together to provide care and preserve the relationships in the family. When it becomes clear that the roles or relationships are suffering to a degree that it has become unpleasant or toxic, something needs to be done. It may be a better solution to hire professional caregivers or other outside services so that the family roles and dynamics can return to normal.

UNDERSTANDING THE LEGALITIES OF CAREGIVING

When our loved ones age and we take on more responsibility, we may feel that we have been given the right to make decisions and take action on their behalf. This can be true to a certain extent, but if they are competent and able to make decisions on their own behalf, our authority may be limited. If they are struggling with maintaining the house and it's falling into disrepair, you have the right to hire a handyman to make repairs. However, if your loved one doesn't want to pay for the repairs, is uncomfortable having workmen in the house, or simply feels the repairs are unnecessary, you cannot force him or her to do so. You can offer to pay or do the work yourself, but you cannot force the issue. Another example is if your loved one lives in a retirement community and has a massive heart attack. You may know that they do not want to be resuscitated, but unless they drew up the proper legal document stating their wishes and the community has it on file, it must call 911, and the emergency responders will take every measure to save the individual's life. You cannot step in and assert that your loved one would prefer to die.

There are five basic documents that every senior should have in place and that are necessary tools for future planning. These forms are available online and are generally accepted if notarized and witnessed, but there may be circumstances where an entity such as a bank or hospital may require a form that has been prepared by an attorney. Often, you can ask local law offices basic questions about forms without charge. You can also contact the attorney general's office to seek advice on whether an online form will suffice or if you should seek an attorney's services to prepare documents.

- **Durable power of attorney.** This grants authority to a designated person or agent to act on behalf of a loved one for specific purposes if your senior is physically or mentally incapacitated.

- **Mental health care power of attorney.** This form appoints someone to make mental health care decisions if a person becomes mentally incapacitated. In some states, only a mental health care power of attorney or a guardian appointed by the court can authorize a person's admission to a mental health care facility for treatment (including dementia with behavioral problems) without his or her consent.

- **Living will (advance directive for health care).** A living will is a legal document that is used to make known an individual's wishes regarding life-prolonging medical treatments. It can also be referred to as an advance directive, a health care directive, or a physician's directive.

- **Health-care power of attorney.** A living will expresses your loved one's medical treatment wishes, but it does not guarantee these wishes will be carried out. The designated health-care power of attorney will be authorized to make important medical decisions about care. If your loved one has a massive stroke and there is no hope for recovery, the living will might indicate if any life-sustaining measures were not desired and the health-care power of attorney would give permission to terminate treatment.

- **Last will and testament.** A will is a legal document that specifies how your client's property will be distributed after his death.

Bringing up the subject of legal documents can be uncomfortable or frightening. It may force your loved ones to disclose personal information they don't wish anyone to know, or it may push them to face their mortality. But it can also bring great relief, knowing that their wishes are specified and the proper documents are in place to allow others to ensure they are carried out.

MANAGING YOUR LOVED ONE'S NEEDS

Being the caregiver of an older person is a complex task. You may find yourself serving in many different roles to meet their needs, not only the expected ones like cook, chauffer, and housekeeper, but also more skilled positions, including nurse, accountant, and counselor, to name a few. Most caregivers receive little or no training to prepare them for the responsibilities they now face. Many find themselves overwhelmed and wonder if there are certain priorities they need to focus on. Fortunately, you don't have to be an expert in order to be a good caregiver. You just need some guidance in what demands can be expected and how to proceed in managing them.

Aside from the basic caregiving requirements such as assisting someone you love with shopping, cooking, and cleaning, it's likely your role will evolve into providing advice and assistance with much deeper issues. The following sections will address these complicated matters and help you prepare in dealing with them.

Managing Medical Care

As your loved ones get older, they may need help in managing their medical care. Juggling multiple appointments, understanding diagnoses, taking medications properly, and so many more tasks can become overwhelming. As their caregiver, you may begin to assume more responsibility to ensure their medical care is handled properly. Here are some tips that will help you successfully manage their care.

- **Be sensitive to their emotions and feelings.** Reassure your loved ones that your involvement is to help them remain as independent as possible while ensuring their medical needs are managed efficiently and accurately.

- **Consider a universal medical record.** This is a tool that will help organize and manage your loved one's care. It is a service that collects, stores, and organizes all pertinent medical information, like prescriptions and doctor's notes, all in one record. With permission, the record can be accessed by health care providers and ensures that all information is up-to-date and that care decisions are not redundant or harmful. Memberships are available through organizations like Pinnacle Care at www.pinnaclecare.com.

- **Obtain authorization for the release of information.** Have your loved one complete an authorization form so that health care providers and pharmacists can interact with you on his or her behalf.

- **Attend as many appointments as possible.** If your loved one is receptive, accompany him or her on as many medical appointments as possible. Information being passed down the pipeline can easily be distorted or misunderstood.

Handling Finances

Money is perhaps the most delicate issue of all and the one most likely to cause great stress and a significant shift in relationships. Your loved ones probably taught you all about handling money, and now they are being told they can no longer be responsible for their finances and that they have to trust you to do it for them.

Many families discover their loved ones should no longer manage their own money after finding that they had not paid bills, were overdrawn, had given the money to scam artists, or were taken advantage of in some other way. According to research by Harvard University economist David Laibson and his colleagues, the typical person's ability to make astute financial decisions peaks at about age 53, then wanes with each passing year; another study found that investing ability takes a steep drop after age 70.

Whether taking over your loved one's finances needs to happen now or you want to prepare for the possibility down the road, these steps will help you begin the process.

- **Plan for the difficult discussion.** Make sure you've correctly identified areas of concern and have a plan on how you are going to help your loved ones manage their money. Unless they are cognitively impaired, involve them as much as possible so they can have a sense of control and trust in your involvement.

- **Document your authority.** Locate any documents, such as the durable power of attorney or living will, that give you the legal right to act on behalf of your loved one. You may have to provide copies to financial institutions or businesses to acknowledge your authority. Ask to be put on your loved one's bank account. If your loved one is not competent, you may have to seek guardianship and become a conservator.

- **Locate all financial accounts and documents.** Ask your loved ones for a listing of all bank accounts, investments, and creditors. You may have to do some serious investigative work. Scan their tax returns and speak with professionals they've worked with, like an accountant, attorney, or financial advisor. Gather up anything that will give you a road map to their finances.

- **Start with balancing the checkbook and move on to paying the bills.** Chances are your loved ones would be more comfortable turning the finances over to you if you start out slowly. Helping them balance the checkbook is a less

threatening place to start. You can then ease into assisting
them with paying the monthly bills. Over time, they will
likely become comfortable enough to allow you to start
managing more of their finances.

- **Seek outside help with larger investments.** Consider using
a financial advisor if your loved ones have a large estate that
includes investments and retirement accounts. If they already
have a relationship with a professional, ask to be introduced.
If not, you may want to hire one.

- **Keep track of your actions.** Because the elderly are sometimes victimized, it's in your best interest and theirs to document your actions. Keep copies of all receipts, payments,
and statements—anything that can verify the legitimacy of
your actions.

Managing the Costs of Care

Ideally, your loved one has bought a long-term care policy and saved
for any future care needs, but often this is not the case. Not everyone has prepared financially, and money will be an issue when making
decisions.

Your loved one's needs may cost a significant amount of money, and
you may be the one who has to figure out how to pay for them. Many
families find that they have to personally supplement these expenses,
which can be financially painful for them. In Chapter 6, we will discuss in detail how to pay for the care and resources for those in need
of financial assistance. For now, there are some actions you can take to
ensure you are keeping expenses under control.

- **Enlist volunteers whenever possible.** Research local eldercare volunteer services to see if some of the care needs can be
met without cost. Many services, like companionship, running errands, and light housekeeping, can be provided free of

charge if your loved one meets criteria such as being house bound or living on a limited income.

- **Interview multiple resources.** Pricing can vary greatly, and even if it's a small difference, it can add up to greater savings over a long period of time.

- **Consider hiring a geriatrics case manager.** A geriatrics case manager is a health and human services specialist, such as a social worker, nurse, or gerontologist, who acts as a guide and advocate for those caring for an aging loved one. This professional can assist in a broad range of issues related to your loved one's well-being and often has extensive knowledge about the costs, quality, and availability of resources in the community.

It is difficult, if not impossible, to estimate how long care may be required. Careful research, planning, and saving can make a difference in whether or not, and for how long, your loved one can afford it. (See Chapter 6.)

Identifying Future Needs

It is not uncommon, and is completely understandable, to focus on whatever needs are demanding attention at a given moment in time. Still, aging and the decline that accompanies it, is ongoing and ever changing. What is needed or works today may be totally different tomorrow. It's wise to consider what those needs might look like over time and have a plan in place to address them. (See Chapter 4.)

Determining Living Arrangements

When asked, most seniors say that their desire is to remain in their own home, no matter how incapacitated or ill they become. Living in their own home represents control and independence, and they

My family is scattered all over the country. I've got four brothers and all of us live too far away to drive and visit Mom on a regular basis. This past winter it was her eightieth birthday and, as a surprise, we all came home to help her celebrate. During our visit, we saw signs that she was struggling with little things around the house like changing light bulbs (most of them were burned out and the house was dark) and cleaning out the cat box. My brothers and I wondered if she was having eye problems, so I took her to the optometrist, and sure enough, she has the beginnings of both macular degeneration and glaucoma.

While there, we went through the house and took care of any repairs that were needed and made sure it was in good shape. We also hired the neighbor's daughter to do some light housekeeping. By the time we left, everything was clean and as good as new.

Several months later, the neighbor called and said that Mom had missed a step and fallen in the front of the house. She was in the hospital. My brothers and I are so upset with ourselves—we knew that her eyes were bad and that the front steps weren't safe for her, but Mom usually went out the back door. She'd been in the front yard because the sprinkler system wasn't working properly, and she was trying to move the hose around to water the grass.

If we'd only thought that when spring came, the yard would need work and Mom would try to do it herself. All we needed to do was hire a yard service at the same time we hired the neighbor's daughter, and she wouldn't have fallen. Unfortunately, Mom's injury required surgery and her ability to get around isn't what it used to be. We just didn't think about what she might need down the road. –*Dale*

may become distressed at the thought of leaving behind their possessions and memories. However, if their health declines and their care needs exceed a level that is safe or affordable for them to remain at home, you may need to help them make other arrangements. It's quite possible that the decision as to where they move will fall on your shoulders.

While the goal may be to help your loved one remain at home, it's wise to research and consider the options that are available if the worst-case scenario comes true. You can explain that while you hope they never have to move, it's in their best interest to learn more about alternative living arrangements. Research communities, request information packages be mailed to you, and perhaps visit for a tour with your loved one. The community may even invite the two of you to have lunch as a guest. Ask your loved one to help you understand what they would prefer if there were no other choice.

Hopefully the move will never have to be made, but by taking a little time to think about the future, you are ensuring that your loved ones will have a say in their future home, if they are not in a position to be in charge when the time comes.

If the decision is reached that your elders should not live in their home any longer, there are other options available. Your choices will be affected by issues such as if family or friends are willing to help, the availability of care communities in their location, and the level of care needed. Here are some possibilities for consideration.

- **Living with family or friends.** Many seniors would find living with family or friends to be their first choice, mainly because they are worried about what it would be like to live in a care community. If there are family members or friends willing to have a senior with care needs move in with them, it can be a wonderful solution. Several considerations need to be addressed before you choose this option, though. Do the caregiver and family understand what will be required to provide care, and are they all willing to participate in that care? Are they capable of providing the level of care needed, as in assisting with toileting or managing medications including injections? How severely will having a person with care

When Dad gave up driving, I tried to discuss with him the merits of moving to a retirement community where they had transportation included in the monthly rate. He wouldn't even consider it. No matter how much I tried to explain that the community I was thinking about had people who were completely independent living in their own apartments and that it was more like a resort than a place for old people, he said no and asked me not to bring it up again.

I was disappointed, because I knew that giving up the keys [to the car] was just the first of many things that would start to happen as he grew older. I was still working, so taking time off to drive him to appointments and on errands was a burden to me.

Three weeks ago, Dad had a stroke. He's in rehabilitation right now and will recover to some degree, but he's going to need assistance with many of his daily activities, like having somebody assisting him when he showers and helping him dress and undress. They also had to put a feeding tube in, and we aren't sure he will ever eat solid foods again. He will need nursing care to manage the feeding tube.

The community I had wanted him to move to is for independent residents only. They can't provide the level of care he needs. There are only two communities that offer the type of nursing care he needs and that's it. He has no other options and I will have to make the decision for him, choose which belongings will go to his new home, and move everything in prior to his release.

He's angry that this has happened and that he has no control. I wish that I had pushed ahead and done the research on my own. At least I would have known what options were out there and could have avoided the nightmare I've been dealing with this past week. –*Christian*

needs move in to the home disrupt their life and relationships? If you choose to have a loved one live with you, there
are resources available to assist you in providing care. Chapter
5 will discuss these in more detail.

- **Moving to a care community.** Today, there are many differences in the types of communities available to the elderly.
  Depending on what type of care is needed, if any, your loved
  one would have several choices to select from. In Chapter 5,
  we will discuss in detail the different types of communities
  there are, what benefits they offer, and how to make the right
  choice as to which one would be a match to your elder's lifestyle, preferences, and needs.

Helping Your Loved One Cope with Loss and Death

By the time they've reached a certain age, the elderly have likely experienced the death of people they have known. They may have been in the
military and seen the death of comrades during wartime or have lost their
parents and now they are losing friends and spouses. It also would not be
unusual for them to be dealing with more than one loss at the same time.
Because they are facing their own mortality as well, it is understandable
that your loved ones might be struggling with depression and sadness.

The elderly can show their grief in many different ways, including
the following:

- greater levels of physical pain

- loss of interest in life and social interests

- increased use or abuse of substances such as alcohol or tobacco

- decrease in personal care, such as not eating and neglecting
  hygiene

- problems sleeping

You can help your loved ones accept the loss of those they cared for and come to terms with their own death by doing the following things.

- **Remember that dealing with loss and grief has no set time-table.** It will take as long as it takes.

- **Acknowledge their loss.** Encourage them to talk about the person who passed and how it affected their life. Let them know they can talk through anything they are feeling and you will just listen if that's all they want.

- **Listen with compassion and respond genuinely.** It's better to say, *"I can't imagine how you must feel,"* or *"I'm not sure what to say,"* rather than hide your feelings or pretend you understand when you don't.

- **Show concern.** Be honest if you are concerned about their well-being. Let them know you care and ask how you can be supportive.

- **Nurture the habit of living in the moment.** When contemplating their own death, the elderly can spend considerable time thinking about the past. Many focus on past regrets. Help them live in the moment by making sure they aren't alone for extended periods of time, engage in conversations based in the now rather than the past, and plan events or activities for the future. Reinforce how much you enjoy having them in your life and what it is they bring to it, such as wisdom and unconditional love.

- **Suggest creating a legacy.** Creating a legacy can help your loved one celebrate their life and give them comfort that they won't be forgotten when they are gone. Recording an oral history, building a photo album, or writing a family recipe book are just a few examples of how this can be done.

JUGGLING YOUR OWN NEEDS
WITH CAREGIVING

Caring for a loved one can be a full-time job, but when you add in other responsibilities, such as nurturing your relationship, raising children, working, and managing a household, it can be overwhelming. Balancing your life can become difficult, and it can drive you crazy.

The most important rule in caregiving is that you must care for yourself first or you will not be able to care for your loved ones. While you can't stop what is happening to your loved one, there are steps you can take to ensure you remain healthy and balanced.

- **Identify and set boundaries.** Everyone has different tolerances, expectations, and beliefs. It's critical to recognize what is benefitting you and what isn't. For instance, if your loved one uses guilt to control you such as *"If you loved me, you wouldn't go on vacation. What will I do without you?"* it would be in your best interest to tell him you've made the necessary arrangements to care for him while you are gone and that it's necessary to take a break so that you are refreshed and able to continue caring for him.

- **Pinpoint and reduce stress.** Identify what is causing your stress, whether it is taking on too many household chores or agreeing to do things you don't really want to do—like babysitting your sister's children on your day off from your job. You don't have to do it all. Ask for the help you need or say no. And don't feel that you have to explain yourself.

- **Understand you don't have to be perfect.** So what if you haven't put a home cooked meal on the table all week? You've spent the past five days with your mother getting her past a terrible bout of the flu. Too often, stress is self-created. We want to do the best we can and judge ourselves harshly if we aren't perfect. Give yourself a break. You're doing the best you can.

- **Accept what you can't change.** Sometimes we think we are in control when the situation is completely out of our hands, such as when your brother insists on taking dad out for ice cream when dad is lactose intolerant. Ask yourself if and what you can change to help the situation, and remember you don't have to take on every battle. Sometimes the best thing you can do for everyone is to just let it go.

My parents don't ask a lot of me yet, but when they do, it's always an immediate need and I have to drop everything for them. Or at least that's what I've told myself. Whenever the phone rings and I see it's their number, my blood pressure immediately goes up. Usually it's something along the lines of they are out of a medication, need me to have it filled and pick it up for them—today! There have been times that one or the other of them has demanded they need the prescription right now because they haven't taken it for four or five days. I've tried talking to them about letting me know when they only have a few pills left but they haven't listened.

The interesting thing is, I've let them do this to me. There isn't any sound reason why I can't say no, that it will have to wait until tomorrow, or that they will have to make other arrangements to manage their medications. When I finally realized that I was the one who needed to set a boundary and then enforce it, I felt so much better. I sat them down and explained that things had to change and that unless it was a life and death emergency, I might not be able to help them until it was more convenient to me. Then I contacted the pharmacy and set them up on an automatic refill program and delivery service. Why I hadn't thought of that sooner is beyond me.

So far, it's working great. Once they realized I wasn't going to jump anymore, they started planning a little more carefully. *—Alexa*

- **Take action when appropriate.** Identify the problem, list possible solutions, select one, and do it. If it doesn't work, try another solution, and if that still doesn't work, maybe it's best to realize the problem can't be solved right now. You can always try again at another time or move on.

UNDERSTANDING CAREGIVER BURNOUT

If you are not careful about recognizing your capabilities in providing care, setting appropriate boundaries, and committing to taking care of yourself first, you may find that you become a victim of caregiver burnout. This is a state of physical, emotional, and mental exhaustion. Burnout can often result from a dramatic change of attitude and you lose your positive and caring approach to caregiving to one that is negative and uncaring.

Some of the signs of caregiver burnout are the following:

- having less energy than you once had and feeling tired and run down
- catching every bug that's going around
- losing emotional control and overreacting
- thinking it is hopeless or that you are helpless
- feeling resentful
- neglecting or treating roughly the person for whom you're providing care

In addition to the tips mentioned in the previous section on managing your own needs, here are several guidelines that can help you avoid caregiver burnout.

- **Set realistic goals and know your limits.** Accept that you may need help or that you can't provide certain levels of care yourself.

Give yourself credit! You are doing one of the most difficult and important jobs there are. Everyone around you is going to have a suggestion of what you should be doing or how you can do it better. When that happens, ask yourself whether they would be willing to step in and take over. Chances are, the answer is no. You may not do everything perfectly, but you're there, and you're trying. In the long run, that's what counts.

- **Be willing to relinquish control.** Allow others to help, even if you don't feel they are doing it correctly.

- **Take advantage of respite care services.** Respite care provides a temporary break for caregivers. It can be provided in home or as a short-term stay in a nursing home or assisted living facility.

CHAPTER 3

Easing Caregiver Concerns with Proactive Behavior

Whether the role of caregiver was thrust upon you during a crisis or slowly crept up on you, you may find yourself handling it by simply putting out fires as they happen. This approach can cause a great deal of stress, dissatisfaction, and unhappiness for all concerned. It's important to understand that, while you don't have control over everything that can happen, you do have the power over how you will react. When you are resourceful, educated as to your options, and aware of solutions to possible issues, you will feel more confident and in control. This can have a ripple effect, resulting in the person you are caring for feeling more secure and developing a stronger sense of trust in the care he or she is receiving.

Part of becoming a successful caregiver is being proactive, recognizing your strengths and weaknesses, and understanding how they affect your ability to provide care. It also involves insightful planning into the future needs of your loved ones, which will allow you to move forward knowing that, when the time comes, you will have the awareness to reach out for help if or when it's needed.

RECOGNIZING THE EARLY
WARNING SIGNS

Trying to plan for every change and possible crisis is overwhelming. It is not uncommon to focus on whatever needs are demanding attention at a given moment. Still, aging and the decline that accompanies it are ongoing and ever changing, and you can't predict every possible scenario. What is needed or works today may be totally different tomorrow. The best you can do is consider what those needs might look like over time and have a plan in place to address them, as well as heightening your awareness of your loved one's capabilities, regularly assessing his or her needs, and continually updating your plans for responding to these changes if they occur.

A great way to take charge of the information you need to accumulate, monitor, and access is to buy a large binder or to create a file on your computer where, over time, you can track issues or concerns and see a pattern of decline. In this document, you can create a reference section with resources that would provide services like in-home care agencies, home and yard care providers, and senior transport companies. You can also record your thoughts or decisions with dates for action. This information is meant to be used as a guideline but to remain fluid and easily updated.

Developing your watchfulness, staying alert, and acting proactively will help ensure that your loved one can remain as independent as possible and possibly minimize your level of caregiving. One key to being able to accomplish this is to break down the overall picture into separate areas such as physical decline and mental decline.

Evaluating Physical Decline

Physical decline is often the easiest change to identify. You can see how difficult it is for your senior to open jars with hands swollen from arthritis or how challenging climbing stairs has become even with the aid of a cane. As you begin to notice these changes, it is the right time to take a look around the home and think about what potential problems your elder may soon experience as things progress. There are some key issues to consider when evaluating physical decline, keeping in mind that each senior is different and that your evaluation can include anything that catches your attention.

- **Home and yard issues.** It is important to regularly assess the safety of the home and how well your loved one is maintaining it. Initially, the solution may be as simple as hiring cleaning and yard services, but as needs increase, other issues such as accessibility, comfort, and safety will demand attention. If you are unsure about or uncomfortable with evaluating the home yourself, there are organizations that will visit, identify potential problems, offer solutions, and modify the home to address the senior's life changes. Search for keywords on the Internet such as "certified aging in place specialists" or "home modifications for the elderly" to identify local businesses providing this service.

- **Mobility issues.** It's likely that, over time, your senior will lose some mobility. They will begin to stumble, may need a cane, or even require a walker or a wheelchair. Here are some questions to give you an idea of what you should be considering.

  ✓ How safely can your loved one navigate the home alone?

  ✓ Will the home accommodate mobility equipment?

  ✓ Are there stairs? If so, should a chair lift be installed or a bath be built downstairs?

- **Bathroom issues.** Bathrooms can be one of the most dangerous rooms in the house for seniors. You might ask yourself certain questions.

  ✓ Is the bathroom safe, or is it a danger zone for potential accidents?

   ✓ It is better to install grab bars, raise the toilets, switch out
the tub for a walk-in shower, or remove bath mats and
install carpet than to wait for a fall?

- **Personal care issues.** Though there are far too many concerns to address them all, here are some questions you should
be asking yourself when monitoring your senior.

   ✓ How long will your loved one be able to shop and cook
without assistance? Should you hire an aide to help?

   ✓ Your senior is wearing the same clothes day after day. Is
the top-load washer and dryer becoming difficult to use?
Should you switch to front loaders or ask the housecle10-
ers if they would be willing to do laundry in addition to
cleaning?

   ✓ Your loved one has had several toileting accidents and has
refused to use protective underwear. How will you handle
these accidents when they become regular occurrences?

- **Pet issues.** You may joke that your senior loves the dog more
than he or she loves you, but it may be true—the dog is an
important part of your loved one's overall happiness. Perhaps
you have noticed that your older person is having a harder
and harder time giving the dog the exercise it really needs
and sometimes forgets to put out fresh water or that the dog
is very young and will probably outlive your elder. Your loved
one worries about what will happen to the dog in that cir-
cumstance. Here are some questions to consider.

   ✓ How long can your loved one care for Fido without help?

   ✓ Who will provide help when it is needed?

   ✓ What will you do with the dog after your senior is gone?

As you can see, the list of foreseeable issues with your loved one's
physical needs can be endless. Do the best you can to be alert to

changes and to be prepared for the future. By researching and documenting any resources or modifications that will be helpful when that need arises, you will greatly reduce the worry and stress of wondering what you'll do when it happens.

Evaluating Mental Decline

Recognizing mental decline can be much more vague and difficult. Perhaps your mother forgot to take her medications this morning. Did she forget because her memory is slipping or was she interrupted and just didn't think afterward? It's possible that it was normal forgetfulness, but if there is a consistent pattern or you see other signs of memory issues, it could point toward a more serious condition. Often with mental decline, it takes time to see these patterns.

Mild cognitive impairment (MCI) can cause changes that are noticeable to the individuals experiencing them or to other people but may not be severe enough to interfere with daily life. Those experiencing MCI may forget information once easily recalled, such as appointments or events, and may also find that their ability to make sound decisions or to follow a series of steps to complete a task are more difficult. Not all people with MCI will get worse, and sometimes they can even get better.

Having an evaluation by a medical professional is the first step toward eliminating more serious conditions, such as dementia, but there are signs you can watch for in order to monitor a worsening of symptoms. This involves asking a variety of questions.

- How often is he or she forgetting things?

- Is your loved one forgetting important appointments or events?

- Is your senior increasingly overwhelmed by making decisions, planning steps, or following instructions?

- Is he or she getting lost or confused in familiar surroundings?

- Is your older person losing his or her train of thought or finding it difficult to follow conversations?

- Is he or she becoming more impulsive or showing increasingly poor judgment?

- Is your loved one able to recognize danger and can he or she respond appropriately?

- Does your senior pose a danger to anyone else?

IDENTIFYING STAGES OF DEMENTIA

The changes that occur with dementia are subtle and can happen over such a long period of time that families often have no idea what stage their loved one is at. They can also worry a great deal over whether it is dementia or normal age-related cognitive decline.

Aside from visiting a doctor regularly with your loved one to assess his or her mental decline, you may be able to identify the phase of dementia if you understand the symptoms of the different stages. You may discover during the assessment process that your loved one is more advanced than you realized.

It is important to distinguish between delirium and dementia. Delirium, often confused with dementia, is a state of cognitive impairment and confusion, disorientation, and memory loss that is usually the result of an illness. The delirious person may not be alert and can be drowsy, semicomatose, or comatose. Symptoms occur rapidly, rather than over a period of time. Delirium is usually caused by a medical condition such as urinary tract infection, heart failure, liver failure, or the use of drugs or alcohol. The condition requires medical attention and, once treated, may completely go away.

On the other hand, dementia is an irreversible state of cognitive impairment and short-term memory loss related to organic brain disease such as Alzheimer's disease, Huntington's disease or Lewy Body disease. Dementia may have a rapid onset with medical conditions such as a stroke, but it is a sustained state, unlike delirium.

My family had always made good-natured fun at the little slips and senior moments my mom had shown during family meals, holidays, and vacations. For us, they were a quirky little part of her personality. Last year, we noticed that Dad was becoming impatient and would snap at her when she'd mix up a story or repeat a question several times. It got to the point that my sisters and I had a huge fight with him, and we didn't talk for a while.

Finally, my dad broke the ice and asked if we would go with them to a doctor's appointment. He wanted it to be a family appointment and wanted all of our input. He was worried that Mom had Alzheimer's disease. We were shocked that he would even say such a thing. Mom was still taking care of him—or so we thought. At the appointment, the doctor did some very specific tests and the news was devastating. She did have Alzheimer's and she was in the middle stage approaching late stage. Dad had done a very good job compensating for her and hiding much of what they'd been dealing with.

Now that we know, we are taking turns visiting almost every day and helping as much as we can. We will have to make some decisions soon, as we can tell that Dad is becoming worn down, and we worry that Mom may start wandering. I still can't get over the fact that they hid it from us for so long and that nobody saw anything. It just shocks me. *–April*

If you suspect that your loved one has dementia, the following information will identify symptoms you can expect at different stages. It is not, however, meant to replace any diagnoses from your doctor and other experts.

Early dementia may be indicated by the following symptoms:

- recent memory loss, which begins to affect normal function
- confusion

- loss of spontaneity, spark, or zest for life; depression may also be present
- loss of initiative, an inability to start anything
- mood/personality changes, anxiousness about symptoms, keeping to oneself
- poor judgment, bad decision making
- taking longer with routine chores
- trouble handling money/paying bills

Moderate dementia may be suggested by the following:

- increasing memory loss and confusion, shorter attention span
- problems recognizing close friends/family
- repetitive statement/movements
- restlessness, especially in late afternoon or night ("sun downing")
- occasional muscle twitches or jerking
- perceptual-motor problems
- problems organizing thoughts or thinking logically
- difficulty finding the right words; making up stories to fill in the blanks
- problems with reading, writing and numbers
- behavior that may be suspicious, irritable, nervous, overly emotional, childish, or inappropriate
- a loss of impulse control; won't bathe, trouble dressing, wearing 2–3 layers of clothing

Severe dementia may be identified by the following symptoms:

- inability to recognize family or self

- weight loss, even with a proper diet
- little capacity for self-care
- failure to communicate verbally
- a tendency to put everything in his or her mouth or to touch everything
- powerlessness to control his or her bowel or bladder
- difficulty with seizures, swallowing, or skin breakdown like bed sores and infections

If you are noticing signs but remain unsure or frightened that it might be dementia, mental status testing, which evaluates memory, the ability to solve simple problems, and other thinking skills, can validate your concerns. It will help you understand whether your senior shows the following symptoms:

- Is he aware that he has symptoms?
- Is he oriented to date, time, place, and who he is?
- Can he remember a short list of words, follow instructions, and do simple calculations?

Contact your senior's primary care physician or ask for a referral to an appropriate health care professional for the testing.

SEEING YOUR LOVED ONE IN TODAY'S REALITY

It's quite normal for caregivers to experience a level of denial and see their seniors as they were in younger, more healthy years than as they are today. This is more likely when the attachment is between family members, especially the relationship of parent and child. It can be difficult when someone you love begins to decline, and you find yourself in the position of having to make decisions or to implement change

My dad used to be the biggest football fan ever. As a child, I remember how we couldn't plan anything if there was a game on television or a local high school game we could attend. Everything revolved around the season.

As he got older and mom passed away, he became quite depressed and lost interest in many things he once enjoyed, including football. I think he may have lost some ability to focus on the game and follow it. Once in a while he'd sit with my brother, Bob, or me while we watched a game, but he wouldn't interact or cheer like he did in the past.

Last month, Dad had a stroke and we realized that he would be better off moving in with one of us. The only problem is that Bob lives in Pittsburgh, I am moving to a small town in Nebraska, and Dad lives in Arizona. Bob is insisting that Dad move to Pittsburgh because he will be able to take him to Steelers games. I don't live near any professional teams. I realize this sounds great, but the fact is that Bob travels extensively for his work, and Dad doesn't get along with his wife. He won't be happy there, and I don't think he cares about the football. I believe he would be happier with me in a town where he would be able to walk to the corner for coffee and everyone would know him. Also, I'm retiring and could spend more time with him than Bob.

We've had some arguments over this. Bob is grieving over what's happened to our outgoing, fun father and he doesn't want to let go of that one memory we cherished—watching games together. Dad won't choose between us. He just says he doesn't care. I think I'm going to have to give in and let Dad go with Bob until they both realize what a mistake it was and then Dad can come live with me.

—*Steven*

on your senior's behalf. You may feel anxious over making the right choices and respecting your loved ones with wanting to maintain your relationship with them.

This is admirable, loving, and kind. However, there is a risk that you may be making decisions based on memories rather than what the individual's capabilities are today. As a result, decisions can be inappropriate or can lack proper focus.

It's critical to be able to assess your senior accurately, acknowledge his or her strengths and weaknesses today, and provide the care that is needed now. For instance, you don't want to insist that Mom must have a companion who plays bridge when she hasn't played bridge in 15 years.

TWELVE SIGNS IT'S TIME FOR ASSISTANCE

If you have someone in your life who you believe is struggling and you are unsure if he or she may need care, the following questions will help determine if your concerns are founded or unwarranted. These questions are designed to encourage thought provoking discussions. If you answer yes to one or more, it is time to consider the possibility that your loved ones may need help.

1. *Are they safe?*

   ✓ In the case of an emergency, can they respond appropriately to help themselves or others in danger?

   ✓ Are you noticing that they are making decisions that might not be in their best interests, such as giving money to every charity that sends a request in the mail even though they are overdrawing their account?

   ✓ Are they putting themselves in situations that could be potentially harmful or life threatening?

   ✓ Are you questioning their understanding and reactions to certain discussions or situations?

2. *Are they a fall risk or do they have an unsteady gait?*

   ✓ Does your loved one have a history of falls?

   ✓ Are you anxious watching them move about?

3. *Are they covering up bruising or scrapes from falls?*

   ✓ Is it possible that they have fallen and are afraid to tell you because they have hurt themselves and can't remember what they did?

4. *Do they need help managing their medications?*

   ✓ Are they able to order refills and pick them up or have prescriptions delivered?

   ✓ Are they struggling with taking the medications as directed?

5. *Do they have an increasing need for help with bathing, dressing, or other personal activities of daily living?*

   ✓ Are they struggling to shower on their own?

   ✓ Have they always cared about their looks, but have now stopped properly grooming themselves?

   ✓ Are they wearing several layers of incontinence pads? Are they aware of when they need to use the bathroom? Do they always make it in time?

6. *Are they able to cook, clean, or shop without assistance?*

   ✓ Are they losing or gaining weight?

   ✓ Do you see rotten or expired food in the house?

   ✓ Are they able to grocery shop?

   ✓ Is the house well maintained and clean?

   ✓ Do you smell odors or see filth?

   ✓ Is the house in need of repairs?

7. *Are you noticing severe hygiene problems?*

   ✓ Do they wear the same clothes over and over?

   ✓ Are their clothes dirty?

   ✓ Can you smell unpleasant odors?

8. *Are they able to manage finances?*

   ✓ Is your dad forgetting to make the utility payments on time?

   ✓ Did he forget to subtract the mortgage payment from the account and is now overdrawn?

   ✓ Has your mom given an excessive amount of money to a charity and can't afford to pay for her medications this month?

9. *Are their cognitive skills, such as the ability to reason or make sound judgments, impaired?*

   ✓ Have you noticed that some or all of their decisions might not be in their best interests?

   ✓ Are they putting themselves in situations that could be potentially harmful or life threatening?

10. *Is their short- or long-term memory impaired?*

   ✓ Are they forgetting if they took their medication?

   ✓ Are you worried that they could drive their car or wander off and not know how to safely get back home?

   ✓ Are they under- or overeating because they can't remember when they ate their last meal?

11. *Are they frequently confused or afraid to be alone?*

   ✓ Do they remember that family has been to see them recently?

✓ Are they having visual or auditory hallucinations that frighten them?

✓ Is their living space so large it overwhelms and confuses them?

12. *Are they becoming isolated from social functions?*

✓ Are they declining invitations to family outings, perhaps because it's too hard to follow multiple conversations at the table? Or have they stopped playing cards with friends at the senior center because they can recognize faces but can't remember names and are embarrassed?

✓ Do you feel they are getting enough socialization?

CONSULTING WITH HEALTH CARE PROFESSIONALS

Symptoms—evidence that there is something wrong with the body or mind—can vary widely from physical issues (such as headaches, weight loss, or incontinence) to mental or emotional issues (such as angry outbursts, anxiety, or depression). Sometimes seniors find it difficult to discuss their personal issues with anyone, including their health care professionals. They may see the need to give out personal information as an invasion of privacy or may be too proud, embarrassed, or intimidated to have an open and honest discussion about whatever is troubling them. They may also be in denial as to what is happening.

As a caregiver, it is important to encourage your loved ones to become partners in their care. When they are hesitant to be cooperative or proactive, you will need to become their advocate. This means that you will need to have your elder give permission for the professional to discuss their needs, diagnosis, or treatments/solutions with you on their behalf.

The following will help you identify key information necessary for you to become a strong supporter and to communicate more effectively with any professionals participating in the health of your senior.

- **Familiarize yourself with her insurance.** This includes health, dental, long-term care, and life insurance.

- **Learn as much as you can about her illnesses or other concerns.** Discuss with your loved one what is bothering her. Talk to those providing care or spending time with her, and ask what they see or feel is important to address. Understand as much as possible about her condition, treatments, medications, or medical equipment before appointments, which will give you a head start in discussions with the medical professionals.

- **Be prepared for appointments.** Understand the purpose of the meeting. Is it a routine follow-up or a thorough cognitive evaluation? Do you need certain information with you at the time of the appointment such as a list of medications and previous surgeries? Don't assume the professionals will have it in their file. When making the appointment, ask if there is any documentation you should bring.

- **Understand your loved one's major concerns and goals.** Ask your loved one what she wants to discuss and what she hopes to accomplish. If the dentist has suggested that your 86-year-old mother undergo major dental work to change her bite and to have her teeth whitened, is there a need for her to spend that kind of money, and does she really want to go through that kind of pain and commitment?

- **Prepare a list of issues and questions you would like to discuss.** If there are multiple topics, write them down. It's easy to forget everything that is on your mind if the conversation turns serious or if the amount of information is overwhelming.

- **Speak up and ask questions if you don't understand or if you have concerns.** Don't be embarrassed if you don't comprehend something the doctor, nurse, or other professional tells you. Don't hesitate to tell them if you don't feel they understand what you are saying.

My dad had been having some delicate issues with urinating and other related problems. I felt that there might be something seriously wrong and asked to go to the doctor's appointment with him. At the appointment, he avoided giving any real answers to the doctor's questions, and when I tried to answer for him, he blew up at me. I was so embarrassed and stunned. He refused to discuss it on the way home.

Later that night, I did some research and found that his symptoms could be a sign of prostate cancer. The only reason I knew about the symptoms is that Mom told me he was having small accidents during the day and then up and down all night trying to relieve himself.

I called and scheduled another appointment with the doctor, but this time I left a detailed message with the nurse as to what was happening. When we showed up the next week, the doctor never mentioned my phone call, but he had all the information needed to ask the right questions. Dad still hesitated to give out too much info, but he said enough that the doctor was concerned and ordered tests. It turns out Dad had prostate cancer, but we were lucky and caught it fairly early. I think if I'd left it up to him, he would have ignored the signs until it was too late.
—*Terry*

- **Take notes.** It can be hard to remember everything being presented to you, especially if you are unfamiliar with the information. Take plenty of notes to refer back to once the material or news has had time to settle in your mind.

- **Ask for a private conversation with the health care professional before the joint conversation.** If you feel your senior won't be honest or will play down or avoid what is bothering him or her, then try to talk with the professional privately so you can relay your concerns and give the doctor a chance to quietly observe or ask more probing questions.

COMPLICATED ISSUES FOR FAMILY CAREGIVERS

Most of this chapter is focused on the person you are providing care for, but there are some areas where focusing on your own future is advisable. By giving some thought to these challenges and what they may mean to you, your family, and your loved one, you may avoid some unwanted consequences down the road.

Long-Distance Caregiving

If you are one of more than five million people providing care for someone who lives more than an hour away, being proactive and planning for possible needs and concerns will serve you well.

In the past, aging parents were cared for by their children or other relatives, but the changes to our lifestyles and the fact that families are often scattered all over the country means that more elderly people are living far from their families. The foundation for successfully providing long distance care is to plan ahead and to be organized.

Here are some tips to help you meet your loved one's needs, avoid crisis situations, and maintain sanity for your entire family.

- **Discuss with your senior what his or her needs are and explain how accepting help will ease your concerns.** Our elders often worry about being a burden, so letting them know how much this will help you can be the key to gaining their acceptance.

- **Use the information from the previous sections of this chapter to create a baseline.** When visiting, you can record and monitor any issues or decline you notice and create a record to look back on and identify important changes.

- **When visiting, take time to meet important people in your loved one's life, such as neighbors, doctors, pharmacist, and friends.** Create a support system by asking for contact information and give them yours so that if there is an emergency, you can be reached and action can be taken. Then stay in touch!

- **Make sure you know where all important documents are kept and make copies for yourself.** Chances are you will need to provide this information more than once to organizations or professionals like banks, health care professionals, lawyers, and pharmacists.

- **Organize other information.** Keep a file with medical records, prescriptions, and important contacts—anything pertaining to your loved one's overall health and well-being. This will be handy if you need to verify or provide this information quickly.

- **Familiarize yourself with local services for the elderly in the area.** Your loved ones may not need help now, but if or when they do, you will have resources to turn to at a moment's notice.

- **Develop specific routines and questions to gauge your senior's capabilities.** For instance, set up a specific day and time you talk on the phone. Create a list of questions you ask each time and see if there are any unusual responses indicating struggles or mental/physical decline.

- **Recognize when you need professional help managing the situation.** If you find yourself wondering if you are doing enough or feeling that it's too much for you, hire help. Find a geriatrics case manager to monitor your senior and put the necessary resources in place. Having someone local that will report to you and act on your and your loved one's behalf can relieve a great deal of pressure and give everyone peace of mind.

My cousin and I live on opposite sides of the country. I am his only living relative and we are both in our eighties. He lives in a nursing home, and I've always felt so guilty that I can't travel to visit him. I know that there have been some issues with the way he says he's treated and he's lonely.

I heard of a woman who offers the service of visiting with the elderly and reporting back to the family what she observes and if she has any concerns. She will even run errands like buying clothes or spend extra time with him on his birthday and more. I hired her to visit twice a month and my cousin loves her. Her visits are the highlight of his week and I know that I can call and ask for anything I need. Also, her reports clear up any issues pertaining to his moods, the care he receives, or other concerns.

It really gives me a peace of mind to know that I have a local set of eyes and ears to look out for my cousin. *–Betty*

Difficulties of the Sandwich Generation

If you find yourself caring for your elderly parents, still raising children, and searching for enough time to nurture your relationship and manage the house, you are part of the "sandwich generation." Trying to do it all can push you to the breaking point. When you realize that you're not handling all these responsibilities very well, you may end up feeling incompetent, hopeless, or demoralized. Getting yourself and your family organized can help you relieve the stress of caregiving now and into the future. Here are some suggestions to start regaining control.

- **Organization, logistics, and time management are a must.** This will require a great deal of time commitment. You probably already feel as though you are being torn in too many different directions before adding on the care of your aging loved one. It is imperative that you organize your time in minutes, hours, days, and weeks. Keep a calendar where everyone can see what time is already committed and can record new events, chores, and even personal time set aside to relax and recharge.

- **Self-care will become even more critical.** You must remember to think about yourself once in a while and do things that will renew and strengthen your ability to manage it all. Schedule date nights with your spouse, take a yoga class once a week, get up before anyone else and walk your neighborhood—anything that gives you a chance to take a breath, relax, and reconnect with yourself.

- **Think of your children first.** While in the midst of eldercare, you may not realize how essential it is to think of your kids first. Dr. Barry Jacobs, PsyD, a family therapist who specializes in issues related to family caregiving and the director of Behavioral Sciences at the Crozer-Keystone Family Medicine Residency Program in Springfield, Pennsylvania, stresses, "A caregiver's first responsibility is to her children, not to her parent." The key to doing this is clear communication with your senior about priorities and with the kids as to how they feel about the caregiving situation and how they might help. With this level of communication, your children will learn lessons about family values, sacrifice, and empathy.

- **If you have siblings, cousins, or other family members who can help, keep them updated and included in the care.** Schedule regular meetings to discuss the current situation and how everyone can pitch in. These meetings can occur over the phone, but it would be more ideal if they happen in person. Meeting face to face allows the participants to see and feel real emotion and the need for help. It's much harder to ignore that one family member who is doing the majority of work when that person is sitting in front of you with dark under eye circles and the phone is ringing off the hook from his or her kids checking in.

- **Ask for help, and don't feel guilty.** You should never feel guilty asking for support whether it's from family or professional caregivers. Asking for help before you are desperate will make this time of life more rewarding and pleasurable for everyone involved.

Is Your Own Retirement Suffering?

It's a mistake to dive head on into the role of caregiver without giving any thought as to how that decision might affect your retirement. Some people will quit their jobs or reduce their hours, and others will spend their own money on providing resources for someone they love. It's important that while trying to do what you might consider right and decent, you don't jeopardize your own financial future and retirement.

Here are steps you can take to minimize any effect caregiving will have on your future.

- **Reconsider any thoughts of quitting your job.** The long-term financial consequences of losing your wages can be far greater than you anticipated. A 2011 MetLife study shows that the loss of total wages, Social Security, and pension accounts for a caregiver over 50 leaving a job early averaged $303,880.

- **Consider taking family medical leave instead.** If the caregiving situation is severe and you qualify, you will be able to take 12 weeks a year of unpaid leave and can return to your position and benefits afterward.

- **Resist the urge to use your savings to pay for care.** Don't jeopardize your future by spending your life savings on a loved one's care. Investigate any resources available to your elder, such as state Medicaid programs, the VA Aid and Disability Benefit, long-term care benefits—even selling or mortgaging your loved one's property to pay for care.

- **Adopt a detached financial approach to providing financial support.** In order to protect yourself, your immediate family, and your own financial future, you may need to say "no" to your parents. Set realistic financial expectations and specify clear terms for providing help such as how much and for how long you will provide support.

If you feel guilty about not providing financial support to your loved one, consider this—you don't want to put your own children in this same situation when you are older and need care. By protecting your retirement, you are protecting them as well.

CAREGIVER SURVIVAL TIP

While you are busy planning and preparing for your duties as a caregiver, remember to plan ahead for some serious quality down time for yourself. Arrange for a vacation or at least a very long weekend several times a year. Find someone to cover for you or make arrangements for your loved one to stay at a community that provides respite care and instruct them not to bother you unless it's a life or death emergency. Then turn the phone off and only check it or your e-mail once or twice a day. Yes, caregiving is a job, but planning ahead and scheduling time to recharge will make you a better caregiver in the long run.

CHAPTER 4

Nurturing Your Loved One's Mind, Body, and Spirit

One of the challenges faced when a loved one is declining is recognizing that simply meeting his or her physical needs may not be enough. There is a definite connection between the mind, body, and spirit, and if all three aren't being nurtured, then the care provided at one level may not be sufficient to create the highest quality of life possible. Not only does an individual's physical care need to be managed, but consideration must be given to that person's mental and emotional needs, as well as offering nourishment for the spirit. All three areas must be cared for as a whole in order to enhance an individual's life—creating as much well-being and zest for life as possible, depending on the circumstances.

Yes, it's a lot to consider, but it doesn't have to be overwhelming. Breaking these needs into three components, understanding what is happening in each, and then deciding on approaches to address specific issues will help keep all the requirements in perspective.

THE MIND: UNDERSTANDING CHANGES
IN YOUR LOVED ONE'S BRAIN

As we age, there are normal changes to the brain that take place. In our early twenties and thirties, the changes can be subtle—perhaps a slight forgetfulness after a particularly hectic workweek or an inability to sleep due to the presence of a newborn baby. By age forty and into our fifties, the changes increase and we may experience more instances of forgetfulness—like forgetting people's names, or why we walked into a room, or what item we wanted to find when we got there. Sadly, some perfectly healthy minds will develop a nagging fear that this could be an early warning sign for Alzheimer's disease and become unnecessarily worried. It can be equally distressing when observing these moments in an aging loved one. The best way to handle these changes is to understand what is normal, explore what the underlying causes of the problem may be, and then determine what, if anything, can be done about it.

What can lead to forgetfulness? Some of the factors might include the following:

- normal brain shrinkage during the aging process

- stress

- anxiety

- depression

- side effects from medication

- medical conditions, including thyroid imbalance, and infections like HIV, tuberculosis, and syphilis

- chronic low-level inflammation of the brain

- declining hormone levels

- dehydration

- poor nutrition

- vitamin B12 deficiency

- excessive use of alcohol or tobacco and drug abuse

There can be many reasons for the changes aside from a serious medical condition. The best way to handle a loved one's fears is to learn how to determine if it's something to be worried about, if anything can be done to improve the mind, and when to seek professional help.

Reducing Those Awkward Senior Moments

Senior moments—those embarrassing seconds when saying hello to someone but being unable to recall a familiar person's name, the dreadful moment when that PIN number at the ATM just won't come, or the frustration over standing in the aisle at the store and having no idea why—can happen to anyone. Most of us laugh about these experiences after the fact, but there are times where they cause genuine concern, especially when they happen to our aging loved ones.

Memory lapses can be frustrating and irritating. The good news is that managing the environment or situation may help reduce the number of times or the degree of forgetfulness the elderly experience. Here are some strategies for reducing senior moments.

- **Reduce the number of environmental distractions.** If your loved one appears to struggle with confusion and forgetfulness during conversations, find ways to reduce the surrounding distractions—turn the television or radio off, choose a more quiet and intimate setting rather than an active restaurant, or provide a private sitting area at a family gathering for visiting.

- **Do one thing at a time.** Encourage your loved ones to focus on one thing at a time and complete each task before moving on to another. For instance, don't hand them their medications while asking if they let the dog out. Multitasking can be confusing for many seniors, and this will help cement the thought or action in their memory.

- **Create everyday routines.** Everyday routines give your loved ones a sense of stability and reduce stress. Set up a schedule for normal daily activities such as taking medications, feeding the pets, checking in with family members, and eating meals. This will also assist you in understanding if something may be wrong, such as when they don't pick up the phone and you know they are awake and should have had breakfast by now.

- **Use reminders and calendars.** The practice of writing down thoughts or information provides security and relief for forgetful minds. Place notepads and pens throughout your loved one's home so he can record important ideas before they slip his mind. Record appointments or special dates on a calendar so he can anticipate and prepare for outings and meaningful events. Or, using large print, write down important names and phone numbers he can call in case of emergencies.

- **Take on fewer activities or commitments.** Seniors can experience forgetfulness, confusion, frustration, and exhaustion if they are overscheduled or overstimulated. Don't schedule everything in one day—a trip to the doctor's office, lunch out, and then getting a haircut may be too much. Choose one or two errands to run, or select just one event at a time so that your loved one can absorb the experience and remember it.

- **Follow the guidelines for a healthy lifestyle.** Encourage your loved ones to eat a healthy diet. If they always reach for processed or fast foods, consider a food delivery service such as Meals on Wheels or preparing dishes ahead of time and freezing them. Make sure there is always plenty of water and other liquids on hand so they can stay hydrated. Buy

them a large cup (32 oz.) with a lid and straw and tell them
to drink two a day. Monitor how much they are sleeping
and, if need be, ask the doctor for medication to help them
sleep through the night. Finally, encourage your loved one to
move as much as they are capable of, whether it's gardening,
walking, or anything else that keeps them from becoming
sedentary. These suggestions will help keep the brain healthy
and boost memory.

Knowing When Memory Lapses Are Normal And When You Should Worry

Although many memory lapses are often just minor annoyances, concerns such as regular confusion or changes in personality or behavior
can signify a deeper problem. As we grow older, it is normal to forget where we put things or to recall someone's name, but when does
memory loss indicate something more serious like dementia?

When observing your loved one, there are key symptoms that indicate cognitive impairment or the early stages of dementia.

- **Repeatedly forgetting names, dates, or incidents.** Anyone
  can forget a person or an event from time to time, but someone with early dementia might repeatedly forget names and
  incidents.

- **Prompting or time doesn't help.** With normal forgetfulness,
  your loved ones may forget information, but when given a
  prompt they might quickly recover or, over time, remember
  the information on their own. However, with serious memory loss, prompting and time have a minor or no effect on
  the memory.

- **Forgetting how to use everyday objects or words.** With
  dementia, it is common for the elderly to forget simple words
  or to use word substitutes that make communication difficult.

They may also misuse or misplace objects. For instance, trying to eat body lotion or leaving the phone in the refrigerator are strong indicators of dementia.

- **Loss of orientation.** If your loved ones become lost in familiar places, don't know what day or time it is, or forget who they are or who family and friends are, they are no longer considered oriented, which is also a strong sign of cognitive decline.

- **Asking the same questions over and over again.** A person with mild forgetfulness should retain information for a reasonable period of time. However, someone with dementia will not be able to make a new memory and will keep repeating the question. The memory simply doesn't stick.

- **Unable to follow directions.** If your loved one has dementia, he might lose the ability to understand basic directions like *"Pick up your glass and drink your water."* He will also need prompting and assistance with normal activities such as eating, dressing, and grooming.

- **Unusual changes in personality or behavior.** Changes in personality, like becoming uncharacteristically angry, aggressive, or clingy, can indicate a more serious condition. Behavior and habits may also change. Someone who normally was an early bird and very social or active might start sleeping or watching television all day while ignoring family, friends, and normal interests.

The symptoms of serious memory loss can be broad and subjective. A thorough examination by a health care professional is called for if there's concern that a loved one may be experiencing more than a normal level of forgetfulness. It is possible that symptoms need to be monitored over a period of time to make a diagnosis and to determine the level of severity.

My parents are wonderful. They are both 83 and living in a small townhouse within walking distance of my home. It's an ideal situation in that we see each other all the time, and it makes it easy for me to pop over and help whenever needed.

I had noticed that when we were with other people and Dad was talking about their past or what they've been doing lately, the stories got mixed up or he struggled with details. I'd have to prompt him with little reminders or he'd get frustrated and shut down, refusing to talk anymore. It's been upsetting to Dad and he kept saying that he thought he was getting Alzheimer's.

I decided it was time to take him to the doctor and have an evaluation done to see what was happening. Dr. Burke ran a bunch of neurological tests and Dad passed them with flying colors. So he asked me if Dad could remember the details when I prompted or if he remembered them later after he had a chance to think. The answer was yes. With that information, Dr. Burke reassured us that if Dad was remembering with a little help or time, his memory loss was not serious. He warned us that if it worsened and Dad couldn't remember at all, then we were right to be worried and to bring him in again.

We were all so relieved to learn that this was a normal level of forgetfulness associated with aging and not to worry—just keep helping when he needed it. I learned not to jump to worst case scenarios just because my parents are aging.
—*Daniel*

Defending the Brain from the Damages of Aging

There is good news, though! Just as physical activity will keep our bodies strong, mental activity can keep our minds in shape. Research shows that pursuits that challenge the brain can offer protection against cognitive decline. A variety of activities may defend the brain from the damages of aging, such as the following:

- engaging in a favorite hobby, like painting or knitting

- reading

- playing games that stimulate the thinking process, such as cards or Scrabble, or completing crossword puzzles

- watching the news or talking about current events

- learning to play an instrument

- taking online courses

This is just a small sample of what might help stave off dementia in the elderly. The rewards from learning something new or accomplishing a challenging experience can reap great benefits. Various studies indicate that it is possible that brain cells can grow and learning can improve throughout life if the mind is kept stimulated. Not only will your loved one feel good about staying active and alert, but he or she may also delay any mental decline that might happen otherwise.

THE BODY: UNDERSTANDING WHAT'S HAPPENING PHYSICALLY TO YOUR LOVED ONE

As with the brain, there will be changes to an aging body. Those changes are largely affected by genetics and lifestyle, but overall, most of us will experience a similar process. Much like the mind, the physical decline can sneak up on us, but it's visually apparent, leaving little doubt. And it can be especially shocking to see how much the symptoms worsen over time when you aren't involved in your loved one's care regularly.

While wrinkles and gray hair are the most obvious, there are a number of other changes that occur in most aging adults. Fortunately, an alert caregiver is aware of them and will seek treatment, help, or lifestyle alterations that can assist a loved one in learning ways to deal with the changes and enjoy a happier, healthier life. We will discuss some of the most common physical changes and offer suggestions as to how to deal with them in the sections that follow.

> My mom passed away a year ago. I've been visiting my dad on a regular basis and helping him with minor things around the house and making sure he was getting by OK. Mom took care of the house and him during their marriage and I just wanted to make sure he was eating, taking care of the dog . . . stuff like that. They had been married sixty years when she passed.
>
> One day when I was visiting, he told me that my brother Mike hadn't been around to visit him in a while. I was surprised, because Mike had told me he'd been over that weekend to clean up the yard. I mentioned that to Dad and he quickly said he'd just forgotten.
>
> A few weeks later, Dad called and asked if I was going to take him to the doctor the next day. I told him yes and that I would pick him up in the morning and we'd have breakfast first. Right before I went to bed, the phone rang and it was Dad again. He wanted to know if he had a doctor's appointment and was I going to take him. He'd completely forgotten that we'd talked earlier.
>
> Mike and I are worried that Dad might be developing dementia, but the doctor said it's normal, old-age, short-term memory loss and that we just need to keep an eye on him. We've decided that as long as he knows who he is, who we are, and where he lives, we aren't going to get too upset over it and start making changes. We have committed to one of us calling or stopping by every day to check on him. It's a small town, and it's easy to do. If anything changes too much, we'll just head down that road when we need to.
> —*Carrie*

Hearing Impairment

Loss of hearing is widespread in the elderly. The changes in the ear make certain frequencies, tones, and speech less clear. This can then lead to an elderly person feeling confused, embarrassed, or left out. Hearing loss may be lessened in a variety of ways.

- **Reduce any background noise and face the person directly when speaking to him.** Speak clearly and slowly.

- **Allow the person to see your face.** Facial and hand gestures can aide in communication. Do not eat, drink, or chew gum while speaking.

- **Repeat yourself, if necessary, and be patient.** It may be difficult for an elderly person to hear or understand the total of what was being said immediately. If he appears confused, say it again, and as many times as necessary. Ask him to repeat what was heard to determine if he understood correctly.

- **Visit the doctor.** Most tests are easy and painless. There are many adaptive devices that can assist the elderly in hearing or communicating more effectively such as hearing aids, telephone amplifying devices, assistive listening devices for televisions and radios, and alarms that will vibrate or flash lights to alert a person that someone is at the door or is calling.

Vision Impairment

For the elderly, the loss of eyesight can cause a number of problems as well as safety issues. Those who can't see clearly might be at risk of falling or injuring themselves and can become insecure or afraid. If they can no longer enjoy reading, watching television, or seeing the faces of friends or family, they may feel lonely and isolated. Loss of vision can affect a person in more ways than simply being able to see.

With age, it's normal for night vision and visual sharpness to decline, and glare becomes a larger problem. This can severely impact a person's ability to drive and maintain independence. The chances of developing cataracts, macular degeneration, or glaucoma significantly increase with age, and routine eye exams become more important. Dry eyes are also common in the elderly and can develop into a chronic condition.

Some of the challenges an individual with poor eyesight might encounter include problems with reading smaller print, seeing clearly in dim light or at night, and being able to locate objects. Regular eye exams, early detection, and proactive measures can help deter further decline or assist in a person's ability to see longer. Here are some suggestions for coping with vision loss.

- **Visit the doctor.** A visit to an eye specialist can determine if your aging loved one has any of the serious conditions discussed previously. If she does, there are many solutions that can assist with her eyesight. With a proper diagnosis, specific recommendations can be made like surgery to correct cataracts, injections to slow the progression of macular degeneration, or drops to control eye pressure from glaucoma. Something as simple as glasses or magnifiers and telescopes could also greatly improve your loved one's vision.

- **Ask for large print.** Large print can make all the difference for your aging loved ones to be able to read everyday items. Larger fonts can enable them to continue enjoying their personal freedom by interacting with others through games, managing their own medications, or staying current with world events by reading newspapers or articles. It's surprising how many items can be adapted to large print.

Prescription labels, playing cards, books, and online magazines are just a few examples of what can be printed in a larger font.

- **Use brighter lighting in the house and utilize nightlights.** Insufficient lighting can be dangerous for the elderly, often resulting in injuries from falling, getting sick because they failed to see that food is rotten, or even letting the wrong person through the door. To help your loved one navigate and manage more safely at home, replace light bulbs with a higher wattage. Seventy-five- to one-hundred-watt bulbs can make a big difference. Make sure entries, stairs, hallways, and other darker areas of the home are well lit and use night lights along the path to the bathroom to eliminate the risk of your loved one falling while using the restroom in the middle of the night.

- **Outline steps or ramps with colored tape.** Stairs and changes in elevation can be difficult for an elderly person to see. Using brightly colored tape on the edge of the stairs or at the beginning of a ramp draws attention and alerts the individual that she needs to move cautiously.

- **Use contrasting colors.** It is easier for an elderly person to see what she is looking for if there is a contrast in color. Buy a phone that has highly contrasting numbers, hang bright towels over the white counter or wall, choose colored soaps and lotions, and throw contrasting blankets and pillows on the bed or couch. Anything that will stand out against the background will be easier to find and use.

- **Make sure medications or supplements aren't causing vision problems.** Check with your pharmacist or doctor to ensure that medications and supplements your loved one is using aren't producing side effects that can cause dry eyes or interfere with vision.

Changes in Bones, Muscles, and Joints

Picture an older gentleman shuffling across the street or a woman who has fallen and is crying out for help. These are common images when thinking of the elderly. As we age, there can be significant changes to the structure of the body. Bodies lose bone mass, joints become less flexible and stiffer, and muscles lose their tone or sometimes become rigid. As this happens, we may experience an increase in pain, start falling, and possibly engage in a more sedentary lifestyle because of their effects. These changes are important for a number of reasons.

- **Bones provide shape and support to the body.** As bones become more brittle, they break more easily. A younger person might recover quickly after a minor fall, but for an older person, it might end with a stay in the hospital and result in permanent damage. Also, osteoporosis becomes more of a problem, especially for women. It can result in a loss of height as the spine and the trunk shorten, and a person can become painfully stooped over.

- **Joints allow the body to move.** Without joints, the body would be unable to bend and move. As the joints break down, the elderly can suffer from inflammation and pain, sometimes resulting in minor stiffness or severe arthritis. There may even be deformity as fluid in the joints decreases and cartilage erodes from rubbing together, or the bones may also start to thicken—think of an arthritic hand with swollen knuckles and bent fingers.

- **Muscles provide strength, endurance, and control for the movement of the body.** Both bones and joints need the help of muscles to operate. Without muscles pulling on the joints, the body cannot move on its own. With the loss of muscle mass, strength and endurance will change. Muscles can also become less toned and can sometimes become rigid. Walking may slow down as movement grows more limited and unsteady. Not only do muscles help us move about, but they

Mom has always been very active playing pinochle at the senior center. She goes twice a week, and it's her only socialization other than family. I came over one Tuesday morning to water her lawn, and she was home. I was very surprised because she should have been at the center.

When I asked Mom why she wasn't playing cards, she started crying. She confessed that she'd decided not to go anymore because she was making mistakes reading the cards, and nobody wanted to be her partner anymore. They couldn't win if she couldn't read the cards properly. Mom was devastated.

I stood there and realized that my poor mom wasn't thinking very clearly. She was reacting emotionally. I told her I'd be back in an hour, and I went home to get my computer. When I got back, we searched online for a store that would sell large-print pinochle cards. With an address in hand, I drove her to the store, and we bought a dozen packs of cards. We decided that she would take half of them to the center with her the next day and keep half of them on hand in case they ever needed them down the road. I also bought her a large magnifying glass on a stand that could sit on the table next to the couch. It had a built-in light and she could hold a book, magazine, or paper under it and still use both hands to hold them while reading. It became very clear to me that I needed to start making changes around her house and yard to accommodate her failing eyesight.

The next day, mom was so excited to head out to the center—not only because she was going to be able to continue playing cards, but she felt as though she was helping others who might not admit they were struggling. —*Gina* also enable our heart to beat, our lungs to breathe, and our blood to flow, along with other numerous involuntary bodily functions.

Muscles, bones, and joints support each other and work together to allow the body to move and function. Even if just one element is declining or changing, it can cause stress and complications for the entire body. Here are some steps that can be taken to help prevent these changes or maintain the body once it starts to decline.

- **Make sure your loved one eats a well-balanced diet and stays hydrated.** Eating a healthy diet is important for anyone, but it takes on a particular importance for seniors. Having a well-balanced diet can help maintain bone strength, boost the immune system, and increase energy levels. Adequate hydration, at least 64 ounces of water a day, will help ensure that all parts of the body—like the brain, kidneys, and other organs—are healthy, functioning properly, and supporting the body as a whole.

- **Use supplements to compliment your loved one's diet.** Changes in appetite, as well as the side effects from medications or illness, are just a couple reasons why a healthy diet might not be enough to ensure overall support of the body's bones, joints, and muscles. Supplements can fill in the voids when the proper amount of nutrients cannot be obtained through diet alone.

- **Encourage regular exercise.** Moderate exercise is the best way to build bone mass, relieve joint pain, and strengthen muscles. An exercise program doesn't have to be intense. It simply requires daily movement. Stretching for 10 minutes in the morning, walking as much as possible, performing chair exercises, or practicing yoga or tai chi are perfect examples of exercises appropriate for seniors.

THE SPIRIT: KEEPING YOUR LOVED ONE'S INNER LIGHT SHINING

Most of us understand how critical it is to care for a senior's mind and body, but not everyone understands that the spirit—that vital essence, inner quality, or nature of a person—needs nurturing as well. True, anyone can exist if the physical body functions at a level sufficient to support life. But what quality exists if that person's disposition or frame of mind is in a low or dark place? Sadly, many seniors begin to lose that vital essence as their physical and mental capabilities decline.

Attitudes toward aging can greatly affect the spirit. Those who view aging as a depressing, useless stage preceding death tend to report a lower quality of life than those who view aging as an opportunity to continue learning and understanding more about themselves and others. The latter attitude tends to promote a sense of joy and purpose.

A variety of changes can cause an elderly person's reason for living to diminish.

- **Death of loved ones and friends.** As loved ones and friends begin to pass on, seniors may start to focus on their own mortality. This can cause feelings of sadness and regret over things they wish they had or hadn't done or said, and they now feel it's too late.

- **Failing health.** When a person is feeling ill or realizing that his or her body is no longer responding and performing as it used to, negative feelings can set in. Anger, sadness, or depression can greatly reduce the overall happiness and quality of life.

- **Altered family roles.** As time passes, family roles become altered. The elders who once guided, provided for, and protected the family are now in need of assistance and care themselves. Children begin to take over the positions once

Like most families, my sister and I took care of our parents until their deaths. I'm happy they were able to stay in their home the whole time, but it was so sad to see the spark go out of them during the last few years, especially for my mom after dad died.

I'm so happy that Liz and I were paying attention at the end. Mom was telling us one day that there was no reason for her to be alive any longer. All of her friends were dead and her husband was dead, what was the point? My God! That was so upsetting to hear it so bluntly said. We immediately put our heads together to come up with something to pull her out of this. Mom was healthy and might just live another 5 to 10 years. We didn't want it to be like this.

Finally, Liz and I realized that Mom had always taken care of everyone—her husband and her children always came first. She had nobody to care for now. We were now taking care of her, and she felt useless.

The very next day, my sister and I visited a dog shelter and picked out a tiny white bundle of fluff. She was a little Maltese and Miniature Poodle mix that had been abandoned during the housing crisis. The family had left her in the home, and the realtor found her almost starved to death. When we laid the dog in my mother's arms and told her the story and that she was saving this little girl from being put to sleep, Mom's spark returned instantly. She named her Boo and immediately went to work giving us a list of things she wanted for her new baby.

Boo and my mom were inseparable for the next two years until my mom passed. That little dog gave my mom something to live for. She had a sense of purpose, someone who needed her to take care of them. —*Chloe*

held by their parents, and family dynamics shift. Navigating these changes may be confusing or difficult for all concerned.

- **Reduced income.** Many elderly find themselves forced to live with less money when they retire. They may struggle to afford prescriptions, food, rent, or care. This can create great levels of stress, affecting them physically and emotionally.

- **Loss of independence.** Perhaps even greater than dealing with the changes in their bodies or minds, the loss of independence hits seniors the hardest. Not being able to do the activities that most take for granted, like driving, managing finances, or even showering and dressing by themselves, can create a sense of no longer being in control.

- **Shrinking world.** Many find that their world becomes smaller and smaller as they age. Being unable to drive and get out on their own, family members being too busy to visit, friends or spouses passing away, or health issues such as losing their sight or hearing, can severely limit an elderly person's environment. Loneliness and isolation can easily set in.

Spiritual nourishment can be delivered in many ways. Steven R. Covey, the author of *7 Habits of Highly Effective People*, wrote, "The need to leave a legacy is our spiritual need to have a sense of meaning, purpose, personal congruence, and contribution." A sense of meaning and purpose are two important concepts that can make a person feel like her life is worth living—creating a sense of self-worth, happiness, appreciation, and a higher quality of life overall.

Fortunately, it doesn't have to take drastic measures to turn around a senior's state of mind and help her enjoy life more. Here are some tips that might get her focused on what she still has to live for and not on what she has lost.

- **Celebrate the small stuff.** An attitude of gratitude can greatly improve a senior's zest for life. Rather than focusing on all

You're doing all you can to provide care and help to your elderly loved ones, but it's not easy. There are days that nothing works and frustration sets in. You can get through these moments by doing the following things.

Choose your battles wisely. Consciously decide whether it's worth it to argue details and correct every error. So what if they are getting the specifics of a story wrong or you're frustrated because they think the checkout boy at the grocery store is your old neighbor's son who is now in his fifties? Save your energy for the important challenges, such as when they insist on climbing a ladder to change their own light bulbs, or when you've noticed they are eating food that has mold on it because they can no longer see or smell it. Determine whether something affects their health and safety before making an issue out of it.

Remember that the situation will not last forever. Unless you have a crystal ball, there's no completely accurate way to predict exactly how long a caregiving situation may last. There will be times when it seems as if this is what it will be like for the rest of your life. Please remember that there is always an end, and for most, when that time comes, you will be glad you gave everything you could to help take care of a vulnerable individual.

Forgive yourself. You're only human. You will lose your patience. Take a time out, regroup, and ask for help if you need to step away for a while. Remember—you are doing the best you are capable of doing.

she has lost or what's gone wrong, encourage your senior to take time each day to think about and give thanks for all that's good. Create a gratitude journal and list five things each day that she appreciates. Or, if writing is difficult, recite it verbally. The point is to develop a habit of acknowledging and giving thanks each and every day.

- **Stay connected.** Seeing people face-to-face, talking on the phone, or using e-mail to stay in contact with others can have a significant impact on one's state of mind. Feeling connected to others eases anxiety, loneliness, and depression. Take advantage of local agencies that offer companionship services, senior centers providing meals and activities, or make regular dates with friends and family that don't revolve around going to appointments or running errands.

- **Volunteer.** Giving back is a wonderful way to feel a sense of purpose and give more meaning to a senior's life. It can be a wonderful way to meet new friends while helping those in need. More and more organizations are realizing that the elderly are a great resource for their volunteer needs. Even if mobility is an issue, volunteers might be able to help over the phone or by working from the home.

- **Pursue a hobby or a class.** Suggest that your loved one consider learning a new language or taking up painting— anything that she has always expressed an interest in but never pursued. Engaging the brain and seeking out new challenges will stimulate the mind and create a feeling of accomplishment.

- **Practice faith.** If religion or spiritual practices were always of importance, find ways to allow your loved one to practice her faith. Arrange for transportation to her place of worship, purchase tapes or books for inspiration and guidance, find television programming that fits her belief system, or locate volunteers who will come to the home and practice with your loved one.

* * * * *

Each of these three areas—mind, body, and spirit—are important. But when providing care for the elderly, it is important to embrace the concept of recognizing and caring for all three together to create a well-balanced existence.

CHAPTER 5

Considering Options for Care Needs

As a caregiver, you will likely have to make decisions regarding who will provide care, which type of assistance is best, and what living arrangement would be most appropriate for your elder's needs. You will also likely worry about how your choices will influence him or her physically, emotionally, and psychologically.

Many seniors say that their quality of life is affected when they must ask for help or, worse, move to a care community and give up their independence. They feel they've lost something vital when they can no longer provide and care for themselves. While it's a natural desire to want to see your loved one remain as self-sufficient as possible, it can lead to the problem of not ensuring adequate care.

As you watch your senior move through stages of decline, it's important to familiarize yourself with the care options available and understand how they can facilitate independence while giving you the peace of mind that your loved one is receiving the support he or she needs, and are as safe and as content as can be expected. Options can range from the family providing assistance, to hiring care providers, to moving to a care community. In order to make the most appropriate decisions, you should be asking a variety of questions.

- If I agree to my mother's request to remain in her own home with care brought in, is she still safe when caregivers are not there?

- Will my father get enough social stimulation if he moves in with me, since I work all day and have an active social life of my own?

- Are there benefits I'm not thinking of with moving my loved one to a care community?

The wonderful thing is that there are options, and being armed with an understanding of what each offers can make the decision process so much easier.

THE FIRST OPTION: FAMILY CAREGIVERS

Most care situations begin with a family member stepping in and helping with chores or activities that are becoming too much for your senior to handle, like grocery shopping, cleaning the bathroom, or laundry. However, over time that person may find that so much has been taken on that it's become a full-time job!

Naturally the First Choice, But Is It the Best Choice?

There are many reasons why family members want to assume the role of caregiver.

- You feel you know and understand your loved one's needs better than anyone.

- You're sure your elder will not accept or be comfortable with help from strangers.

- You don't trust others to provide quality care.

- There are issues your family would like to keep private, like behavioral problems or a history of abuse.

- They are your family, and it's your duty to care for them.

While these reasons are understandable, it doesn't mean that family caregivers are the best choice for you, your loved one, or your family. Here are some signs that might indicate a different caregiving solution is called for.

- Health care professionals feel your elder's needs exceed what you are able to provide, such as caring for open wounds or for someone who is completely bed bound.

- You have limited time to provide ongoing care or may not be able to respond promptly in case of an emergency.

- Your home or lifestyle isn't conducive to being a primary caregiver; perhaps your teenage children would need to share a room if Grandma moves in, or you and your spouse both travel extensively for work.

- Your relationship with your loved one is strained and would be an uncomfortable situation for one or both of you.

If you are considering being, or find yourself becoming, the primary caregiver, give serious thought to your elder's needs, your abilities to provide for those needs, and how it will affect the quality of life for all involved.

Not Everyone Is a Natural Caregiver

Most people hope they would be willing to care for a loved one in need, but the reality is that there are people who do not make good caregivers. Not everyone has the personality, skills, or talent to become

I am the oldest in a family of nine children. When I was 15, Dad died in a car accident and mom was left raising and providing for all of us. It was hard on her, and she grew distant and cold. As soon as they could, my siblings left home and moved away. For some reason, I stayed near Mom and now that she requires help, I find myself doing it all and I'm resentful. It's not that Mom was abusive—she just never gave me any tender loving care or showed any interest in my life. My siblings don't help because they live out of state.

It feels like punishment having to care for a mother who didn't nurture me as a child. After counseling, I've learned that the responsibility should not fall on my shoulders alone. I've decided to ask my brothers and sisters for financial help to pay for a caregiver to do the cleaning, shopping, and cooking. There are ways to make sure she is OK without physically or financially doing it myself. *–Connie*

a top-rate musician, politician, or accountant—why should we expect that all family members would make wonderful caregivers? If there is a situation where a family member is expected to provide care and that person is stressed, miserable, or resentful, both the caregiver and the care recipient are going to suffer. Think twice before forcing yourself or another to accept the role of caregiver. Consider the reasons why any person being considered may not be the best choice, learn about other available options, and be understanding when addressing that individual's lack of interest or commitment.

THE ROLE OF A HEALTH CARE ADVOCATE

As a caregiver, if you are insecure or unable to manage medical decisions or information, a health care advocate might be a valuable addition to your resources.

A health care advocate acts as a liaison between health care providers and your loved one. This includes medical personnel, insurance companies, facilities—virtually any person or organization providing health care services. Mary Jo Beardsley, RN and founder of Peace of Mind Professional HealthCare Advocacy, explains that an advocate will assist clients and their families by helping them navigate complex systems to receive optimal care and outcomes. Here are some examples of what those services might look like.

- Coordinate and monitor crisis situations, such as when a client is having chest pains and has been transported to the hospital. This might include the advocate meeting the client and his or her family at the hospital, explaining what is happening, guiding them through their options, sharing in the decision making, and protecting them from procedures that may not be necessary.

- Provide the knowledge needed to make key health care decisions based on your individual goals. The advocate will offer information and advice on insurance, medical procedures, tests, treatments, medications, community resources, and more.

- Assist through all transitions of care by managing the components of that care so that no information is lost or misunderstood. For example, if your senior suffered a stroke and is moved from the hospital to a rehabilitation center for occupational, speech, or physical therapy, the advocate will confirm that all the records are properly transferred with your loved one and that the staff at the rehabilitation center is aware of any specific instructions or concerns.

- Assist with placement into rehabilitation centers, assisted living, nursing homes, palliative, or hospice care facilities.

- Screen, arrange, and monitor in-home health care or other services.

- Accompany your loved one to visits with his or her health care provider.

- Coordinate resources like transportation services or home health care agencies.

- Assist in reviewing medical billing and interpreting insurance policies.

On average, rates for a health care advocate range from $75 to $250 per hour.

The benefits of having a health care advocate can be immeasurable because the advocate will allow you and your loved one to focus on obtaining and maintaining optimal health without having to worry about complicated details.

CHOOSING BETWEEN PROFESSIONAL HOME HEALTH CARE AGENCIES AND PRIVATE CAREGIVERS

There will be circumstances when caregivers decide they need to seek additional help. Perhaps they've realized they are missing too much work and their job is at risk, or they are ill or incapacitated, or the level of care required exceeds their capabilities.

Ralph Fern, owner of Homewatch Caregivers in Scottsdale, Arizona, offers valuable information concerning the decision as to whom to hire as a care provider, as well as on how to interview potential agencies and private individuals.

Professional Home Health Care Agencies

Professional agencies can be broken down into two separate types of care providers—*home health care* and *home care*. Both agencies will supply private caregivers (also known as home health or home care aides) who will assist your loved at home, but there are distinct differences between the types of care they deliver.

Home health care agencies provide skilled medical care in the home. Home health care may be necessary after a doctor's visit, when it is noticed there is a need for physical therapy or there are problems recovering from an illness, or it could also follow a stay in the hospital when ongoing treatment is required. Services are provided by medical professionals such as nurses, doctors, and therapists or, at times, home health aides like certified nursing assistants. Home health aides are supervised by other medical professionals. Aides may provide basic health services such as checking vitals, administering medications, assisting with medical equipment, and changing bandages. Overall, home health care services include the following:

- skilled nursing

- caring for wounds

- pain and prescription management

- at-home physical therapy

- recovery from an illness or other health problem

Nonmedical home care services are provided by home care aides who visit and support your elder while assisting with his or her normal day-to-day activities, such as the following:

- bathing and dressing

- moving around and remaining safe while getting in and out of the shower, bed, or chair

- helping with household chores such as light cleaning, vacuuming, and laundry

- running errands like grocery shopping or picking up prescriptions

- reminding your elder when to take medications

- providing companionship for isolated or homebound seniors

Both types of caregivers will help your loved one remain in his or her own home or with you for as long as possible.

Private Caregivers

The third option available to you is to hire a private, non-agency-related individual to act as a caregiver. This might include a retired nurse who wants to work part-time, a former health care agency aide, or some other individual trained and experienced in the health care industry. Many families seek to hire a private caregiver with no affiliation to a home health or home care agency because an independent caregiver often charges less. While this may be financially beneficial, there can be certain consequences or risks to you and your senior if you choose to do so.

Tax Considerations

As an employer, your first responsibility is to verify that the caregiver you hire is legally qualified to work in the United States by requiring the potential employee complete an Employment Eligibility Verification (I-9) Form and reviewing documents showing the employee's identity and employment authorization such as a US Passport, Certificate of US Citizenship, Certificate of Naturalization, or Permanent Resident Card.

You will also need to be responsible for processing, withholding, and paying payroll taxes to the government. In addition, as an employer, you must comply with all federal and state wage and hour laws and regulations as well as paying for state unemployment insurance.

Workers' Compensation and Liability Issues

There are additional responsibilities aside from payroll taxes involved in hiring a caregiver who is not an employee of a home health/home care agency. As an employer, you are required to provide worker's compensation. In some states, it is a criminal offense if you do not comply.

Typically, caregiving is an extremely physical job, and the caregiver is particularly at risk for injury if your loved one's needs require substantial exertion such as lifting dead weight, assisting in transferring from a bed or a chair, or providing support while showering or bathing. If your caregiver sustains injuries while performing caregiving duties, you or the individual receiving care may be responsible for medical expenses and disability payments. Typically, homeowner's insurance will not cover a caregiver for an employment-related personal injury.

There is also the liability of your employee possibly injuring another person. If, for example, the caregiver accidentally trips an older friend visiting your senior and that person breaks a hip, or if the caregiver has a car accident while running errands and injures the other driver, you may find yourself subject to a lawsuit if you aren't carrying proper insurance. You can save a lot of financial and emotional stress if you consult with your insurance professional beforehand to identify what types of insurance you may need to protect yourself.

Abuse or Exploitation

Most individuals who become caregivers do so out of a strong desire to help others. But there will always be those who will take advantage of the vulnerable. This is especially easy if your loved one is frail, functionally limited, or has cognitive impairment, and the caregiver is left alone with your senior with little or no supervision.

Abuse and exploitation can take on many forms, such as physical abuse, ignoring boundaries and developing inappropriate relationships, or stealing possessions or money and identity theft. If you are a private employer, it can be challenging to discover any previous issues your new caregiver may have been involved in.

Your first step toward ensuring the applicant is safe to have in your home and caring for your loved one is to ask for references, follow up with phone calls, and conduct a criminal background check. This should alert you to any obvious signs that the applicant has had problems with previous employers.

Next, verify what training the caregiver has received to provide caregiving services. If the person has attended certification programs, ask for copies of the certificates. If the training was on the job, request information on whom you can contact to discuss the applicant's performance and abilities.

Finally, establish boundaries. It is easy for a caregiver to become too familiar with a patient. If the person provides care for any length of time, strong bonds may be formed and both sides may forget what's appropriate and what's not. Draw up an employment contract that states clearly what the job description is and what behaviors or actions will not be acceptable and will result in dismissal.

* * * * *

When faced with making a decision about who will provide caregiving services to your loved one, you need to take into account a variety of questions.

- What type of help is needed: skilled or basic home care?

- Are there any financial or tax implications?

- What is your liability?

- Who will supervise the care?

- Can your loved one alert you if there are any problems regarding his or her care or well-being?

If choosing a private individual, it is advisable to consult with an attorney and an accountant to ensure that all agreements and arrangements meet required safeguards and obligations. It is also responsible to investigate your state's small business laws to make sure you are following all rules and laws.

Interviewing Professional Home Health Care Agencies or Private Caregivers

Once you've made the decision that you need to enlist help, there are specific questions that should be asked in order to ensure that you will be receiving quality assistance. Here are sample questions that should be asked and that will guide you in your interview process.

Interviewing Professional Health Care Agencies

- What are the agency's qualifications and those of its caregivers/aides?

  ✓ Is the agency licensed by the state? (Many states, but not all, require agencies to be licensed and reviewed regularly.)

  ✓ Is it Medicare certified for federal health and safety requirements? If not, why?

  ✓ Does it hire employees or utilize independent contractors?

  ✓ What is its employee screening process? Does the agency run background checks and do fingerprinting?

  ✓ Can it provide references from other professionals it has worked with, like nurses, doctors, discharge planners, and hospitals?

  ✓ Can the agency provide references for the caregivers it would consider for your loved one from others it has provided care for?

- How does the agency ensure quality of care?

  ✓ What credentials does it require from its caregivers?

  ✓ How does it train, supervise, and monitor its caregivers? Do the caregivers receive continuing training or education?

  ✓ Is the agency and its caregivers insured?

- What can you expect in costs and billing?

  ✓ How does the agency handle expenses and billing? Ask for an explanation of all services and fees.

  ✓ Does it accept health insurance or Medicare?

  ✓ Are there any resources that could help pay for care? Does it have payment plans?

- How will you understand the services the agency will provide?

  ✓ Will you receive a written plan of care prior to services?

  ✓ How frequently is the plan updated and what type of information does it contain?

  ✓ Does the agency provide a patient's bill of rights?

  ✓ Does it refer out to specialists like dieticians or physical therapists?

  ✓ Who will provide care for your loved one? Will your senior see the same faces, or will there be a rotating schedule and unknown caregivers coming in to the home?

  ✓ How does the agency handle its caregiver's sick days, vacations, or holidays? Who provides care when the caregiver isn't available?

  ✓ How will its caregivers handle emergencies such as a fall or a heart attack?

  ✓ Does the agency have a plan on how to handle emergencies such as power failure or natural disasters?

  ✓ How does the agency handle requests, questions, or complaints?

Interviewing Private Caregivers

- What training or certifications does the caregiver have? Will the person be willing to attend additional training if you pay for it?

- Given your senior's needs and what would be expected from you, is there anything on your list that is a concern for the caregiver?

- Has the caregiver ever cared for someone with needs similar to those of your loved one? If so, ask for a detailed list of the services or care provided.

- Is the caregiver able to work the hours required?

- Is the caregiver available or flexible to work additional hours in cases of long weekends, respite care so family members can have extended periods away from their loved one, or emergencies?

- Will the caregiver submit to a background check?

- Is the caregiver comfortable with family or friends coming in to the home while the caregiver is working?

- Does the caregiver have a driver's license with a clean record, reliable transportation, and insurance?

- Are there any other responsibilities that will affect the caregiver's ability to honor your schedule, such as other jobs or family commitments?

- Is the caregiver willing to sign a contract that the caregiver will not have guests at the home unless you have given prior approval?

- Is the caregiver willing to sign a contract that the caregiver will not accept money or gifts unless you have given prior approval?

- What does the caregiver expect in terms of vacation or sick days?

- Does the caregiver smoke? This is important if you or your loved one do not want a smoker in the home.

- Given specific scenarios, ask the caregiver how those situations would be handled. For example, what steps would be taken to handle your father if he fell, if your mother had a fever and vomited, or if your loved one was combative?

If you are at a loss as to where to begin searching for a private caregiver, there are organizations such as Care.com that can assist you in finding candidates and running background checks.

PALLIATIVE CARE SERVICES

There is a relatively new resource available to individuals who have a serious medical condition or illness like congestive heart failure, kidney failure, HIV/AIDS, or Parkinson's disease and are in need of a higher level of care but are not ready for end of life hospice care. Palliative care focuses on improving quality of life by providing patients with specialized medical care that will relieve symptoms, such as the following:

- pain

- shortness of breath

- fatigue

- constipation

- nausea

- loss of appetite

- difficulty sleeping

Palliative care can also improve your loved one's ability to tolerate medical treatments and gain strength to carry on with daily life.

Patients and their families face a great deal of stress during an illness and may experience symptoms like fear, anxiety, hopelessness, or depression. Through palliative care, treatments may include counseling, support groups, family meetings, or referrals to mental health providers. Your care provider can also help with practical issues such as explaining complex medical forms or answering insurance questions.

Palliative care promotes a proactive approach to care and is provided through a team that includes a doctor, nurse, social workers, and perhaps other experts such as nutritionists, massage therapists, pharmacists, and spiritual counselors. Your team will work with you and your senior to support your family by not only controlling symptoms but also helping you understand treatment options and goals. Care may

When my mother was diagnosed with breast cancer, she endured chemotherapy and radiation treatments that left her severely nauseated and fatigued. She constantly felt horrible and was in pain from the radiation. She also struggled to understand her treatment and became depressed and afraid of what her future looked like.

Mom has lived with me and my family for the past two years, and I found myself worrying about how we were going to get through all of this. After talking with the case manager, the hospital strongly recommended that she be placed on palliative care to help manage her symptoms during recovery.

I don't know what I would have done without our team. They've been a tremendous support system, and I have more confidence in Mom's ability to fully recover; remain at home; and to live a healthy, happy life. If the worst case happens and the cancer comes back or spreads, I know that we've got people to help us navigate the difficult road ahead. –*Barbara*

be given at any time and at any stage of an individual's illness, from diagnosis on. Moreover, palliative care can be provided in addition to curative care.

Palliative care is offered through organizations like hospitals, hospice, home care agencies, cancer centers, or skilled nursing facilities. If you believe your loved one would benefit from this, speak with his or her doctor and ask if your loved one is a candidate for it.

Care is paid for through personal funds, private insurance, or through programs provided by select hospitals or skilled nursing facilities.

HOSPICE SERVICES

Hospice is a unique health care option available to patients and their families who are faced with a terminal illness. It can be an invaluable resource for families and caregivers who are doing everything possible to tend to their elder in the last stage of life. The surprising fact is that many people don't understand that hospice programs not only provide comfort to an individual during those final days or months when he or she is dying but can also be a tremendous support system for the family and those who are actively involved in their loved one's care.

While most hospices share the same philosophy toward end of life care, their services may differ. Hospice is considered a medical specialty like cardiology, oncology, or pediatrics, so each hospice is its own company and may choose to provide certain services and not others. Barbara Volk-Craft, PhD, MBA, RN and Director of Program Development for Hospice of the Valley in Phoenix, Arizona, explains how many hospice programs operate and how hospice care can benefit you and your loved one.

While the focus will be on making your loved one as comfortable as possible by managing pain and symptoms, hospice teams can assist the family on the more practical side of care, such as bathing your senior, helping with medical equipment, administering medications, providing assistance with paperwork, or finding resources. They also make available invaluable emotional support through grief and spiritual counselors before, during, and after the death of your elder.

Hospice end-of-life care focuses on caring, not curing, and believes that every person has the right to die pain-free and with dignity and that its purpose is to provide the necessary support to do so. Services are primarily brought in to the private home or through hospice acute centers. In some states, services can also be offered in nursing homes, hospitals, and long-term care communities.

To qualify and receive hospice care, your loved one's physician must state that death can be expected within six months. However, nobody can predict when death will actually happen, so this does not mean that care will only be provided for six months; it can be provided as long as the physician and hospice team recertify that your elder's condition continues to remain life limiting. Every sixty days, the doctor will need to reevaluate and state that your senior still qualifies for hospice services.

There are four levels of care provided through hospice.

1. **Routine home care.** This is the most common type of hospice care and includes nursing and home health aide services. Intermittent care will be provided in the home or a long-term care or assisted living facility.

2. **Continuous home care.** This care is provided during a crisis in which your loved one may require continuous nursing care for comfort and relief, also known as palliation or the management of acute medical symptoms. The care is provided in the patient's home or wherever the person lives. In addition to the normal hospice team, your senior could receive up to 24-hour care by a licensed nurse or hospice aide.

3. **Inpatient care.** This care is for pain and symptom management that cannot be provided at home or in another living situation. Care would be provided in a hospital, hospice acute center, or long-term care facility to gain control of the pain or symptoms, after which your elder would typically return home.

4. **Respite care.** This is short-term care provided to your loved one in a hospital, hospice center, or long-term care facility to provide a break in caregiving duties to the caregivers. It is only provided out of home and on an occasional basis.

Your loved one's hospice team would likely consist of a doctor, nurse, social worker, counselor, chaplain, home health aide, and trained volunteers. Some of the services the team can provide include the following:

- managing pain and symptoms
- providing medications, medical supplies, and equipment
- delivering personal care like bathing or grooming
- coordinating services like speech and physical therapy
- teaching family members or other caregivers skills to assist in providing care
- offering bereavement counseling for grief support and education
- giving general support and counseling to family members while their loved one is receiving services

Most hospices are certified through Medicare and must adhere to a core set of services that are available to all patients receiving hospice care. Individual hospices can selectively add to their program with additional services such as massage therapy or pet therapy. Hospice services are provided free of charge, regardless of a person's ability to pay. Hospice care is paid for through the Medicare Hospice Benefit, Medicaid Hospice Benefit, and most private insurance companies. If your senior does not have coverage through these sources, hospice programs will work with you and your loved one to ensure services are delivered.

CARE COMMUNITIES

Although most people will say that their main desire is to remain in their own home or with family as they age, that may not always be the best solution to meeting your elder's needs.

Let me share the story of Karen, who faced the same dilemma so many caregivers face each day, to illustrate how easy it is to ignore the growing signs that a different living arrangement is needed.

Anxiously, I watched my mother rising from the chair. She rocked back and forth, building just enough momentum to propel herself forward and wildly grab for the walker's arms. I couldn't help myself as I mimicked the rocking, silently urging mom onward and praying she'd make it.

Did she lock the wheels? Are her legs strong enough to hold her if she does miraculously make it up? What if she doesn't grab the walker just right? She could fly right over the top and break her neck!

A thousand doubts and questions filled my mind in that second and almost every other second of every day.

For the past six months, I had abandoned my husband and our dream home to move in and watch Mom. Watch her say good-bye to her precious tabby because he was a tripping hazard. Watch her lose 15 pounds in three months because she no longer had an interest in cooking or eating. Watch her style only the front of her hair and spend the day looking like a bird's nest from behind because it was too difficult to stand, hold the mirror, and comb the back of her head at the same time. Each day brought a new awareness that I was watching her disappear.

Mom is a fiercely independent woman with a quick wit and an even quicker temper. A former marine, she was used to barking orders and demanding respect. When I suggested to her that we either have help come in to the home on a daily basis or we take a look at assisted living, Mom would have nothing to do with it. She would stare me down: "I took care of you all those years and now it's your turn." Sadly, I backed down and remained with Mom for six more weeks—six weeks until Thanksgiving, when she took a tumble and broke her back. Upon consulting with the doctors, I was told Mom could not go back home, ever. She needed assisted living and would only be discharged to a care community. I knew we had let the situation go on for too long, and now her life had been turned upside down and her options were severely limited. Without any plans in place or knowledge of communities available, I stress about the journey ahead, unsure how to make it happen or where to begin.

This is a familiar scene across the country—children afraid or unable to convince their loved ones of the merits of assisted living. The tragedy is that the fear and frustration revolves around ignorance and misconceptions. With a proper understanding, assisted living can be a positive, life-enhancing experience.

The Purpose of Assisted Living

Assisted living can be a highly desirable solution for families. It is a bridge for that large gap between being able to live completely on your own and needing skilled nursing care. It allows residents to live as independently as possible while providing as much personal care and support services as needed. The variety of housing options provides an atmosphere suitable for all levels of care—ranging from someone who is completely independent but understands there may be a need for services in the future to a resident suffering from advanced Alzheimer's and needing a secured environment now.

Communities are designed to provide help with the activities of daily living (ADL) such as bathing, grooming, medication management, mobility issues, and more. Usually, residents have had some sort of decline in health and need help performing one or more ADL. They may start out with minimal assistance, and as their needs increase, the support and assistance will increase accordingly.

The Benefits of Assisted Living

When you first consider the possibility of moving your loved one to an assisted living community, it is usually with a sense of finality. Your senior has lost the ability to live alone or with family, and it may seem as if this is the beginning of the end. It's possible you haven't considered the benefits of assisted living aside from the assurance of general care and support.

While every resident and family may experience a different outcome depending on their own personal situation, the following are some of the additional and unexpected benefits your loved one may receive living in a community.

Safety

As most people age, they become frail and the risk of falling increases. Following an accident, younger people might be able to brush themselves off and move on, but the chance of an elderly person suffering a severe injury and ending up in the hospital is high and the consequences can be serious. Accidents may result in not only hospitalization but also disability or even death. One fall can turn into a life-changing event.

Assisted living communities concentrate heavily on the physical safety of their residents. Here are some of the steps taken to prevent falls and injury.

- Staff members are trained on how to properly lift and transfer residents.

- Escort services to meals or activities are available for those still mobile but who are unsteady on their feet.

- Stand-by or full shower assistance can be provided to minimize fall risks in the bathroom.

However, physical safety is not the only focus. Assisted living communities place great emphasis on securing the community from crime or acts of nature. What a great relief for a family or a senior to know they no longer have to worry about safety inside their home and being alone in the case of an intrusion or natural disaster. Common security measures or procedures include the following:

- requiring visitors to check-in before seeing residents

- security guards on staff

- video cameras to monitor the premises

- auxiliary entrances that are locked and require a card key or numeric code to gain access

- emergency plans with procedures for evacuation in case of bad weather, fire, or other emergencies

- routine emergency drills

- regular inspections to ensure the building is up to code

Another safety feature is the protection against potential scam artists or family members that would take advantage of their senior relatives. While no community should handle its residents' finances, a certain level of awareness and monitoring can be provided with regards to who is visiting the resident and the reactions to these visitors. Solicitation and abusive behavior are not tolerated and would be reported to other family members or the proper authorities.

Nutrition

As we age, it's not uncommon for our tastes to change or to lose our appetites. In addition, grocery shopping and cooking can become difficult, if not impossible. Weight loss or lack of nutrition can have serious consequences for anyone who is suffering from health issues or overall decline. Maintaining a healthy weight range is very important for all of us, but it is especially critical for the elderly.

Our dad was complaining of not having any money, but we knew he was bringing in enough to cover his mortgage, living expenses, and then some. For the past year, he increasingly complained that his money was running out, and he couldn't pay for all of his medications.

Dad had always managed his own finances and had done a good job—at least, we thought so. Upon examining his bank accounts, we found payments to credit cards we didn't know existed; several of them were fully maxed out. When questioned, Dad became very angry and defensive and the family decided it was necessary to freeze the cards and investigate further.

Sadly, in Dad's loneliness, he had become susceptible to online advertising from young women looking for men to support them. He had established a long-distance "relationship" with a woman who convinced him that she was his girlfriend and if he would only help her with this or that, it would show how much he loved her. Our father was 85 years old and this woman was 33. He was securing credit cards and adding her onto the account. When she would reach the limit on one card, he would get another for her.

Obviously Dad's judgment was impaired and we started to notice other signs that he was not making sound decisions. We insisted on assisted living, which has strained our relationship with him. However, with the help of the community, his activities on the Internet, phone, and his mail are monitored and his finances are safe. By the way, the "girlfriend" recently broke up with him. *—Ron and Lee*

Too much weight can trigger unwanted side effects, such as the following:

- diabetes, heart disease, and other chronic diseases
- high blood pressure and high cholesterol levels
- stroke
- some forms of cancer
- loss of mental acuity

But too little weight can trigger its own set of problems, such as the following:

- lack of energy or vitality
- slowed healing from illness or surgery
- higher risk for infection, depression, and death

Assisted living communities provide nutritious and appetizing meals for their residents. In larger assisted living communities, it's not uncommon to find restaurant-style dining provided in one or more settings and possibly a bistro for complimentary snacks, newspapers, and socialization. Smaller group homes will feature homemade meals catering to an individual's tastes and preferences. Depending on the community, one to three meals—along with snacks—are provided daily for residents, and special dietary needs for conditions such as diabetes, heart disease, or allergies can be easily accommodated.

For a senior who has stopped preparing meals or is only eating prepackaged food, there is a risk of severe malnutrition and unwanted weight loss. Having balanced and nutritious meals prepared and then being supported with gentle encouragement to eat more frequently will lead to better health. With proper nutrition and hydration, residents often experience an overall improvement in their health within a few months of moving to a community.

Transportation

Many assisted living communities offer transportation within a certain radius. Residents can give up their car keys and remain as mobile and independent as they were behind the wheel. They don't have to feel trapped at home or dependent upon others. Communities offer transportation for a large variety of outings such as the following:

- doctors' appointments
- visits to the beauty salon
- trips to the bank and post office
- shopping
- dining out
- casino outings
- movies or plays

These services are equally as freeing to a family member who has been providing transportation services.

Housekeeping

In assisted living, basic housekeeping is provided regularly. In a private group home, you will see staff cleaning daily, and in the larger assisted living centers, housekeeping will visit weekly or biweekly. Trained staff will also handle maintenance and other not-so-routine tasks such as cleaning out the fridge, washing windows, and changing light bulbs or air filters. Being able to give up the day-to-day responsibilities of managing a home can increase the comfort and safety for older adults. It also frees up their time to enjoy more pleasurable activities.

Laundry

While assisted living communities perform linen service weekly or as needed, residents have the option of continuing to do their main laundry themselves in their own home if appliances are available, or they can pay to have staff take care of their laundry needs. Most communities have communal laundry facilities and many are coin free—all the resident needs to provide is the detergent. It's not uncommon for communities to also offer dry cleaning runs and ironing.

Friends

Communities encourage residents to engage in conversation, social activities, and to develop relationships with other residents and staff. Staff, ambassadors, or welcome committees greet new residents, making sure they aren't alone when they first move in and making sure they have someone to eat and attend activities with until friendships blossom. Even if some seniors struggle in the beginning and avoid social contact, there will be someone there to gently provide encouragement until they come out of their shell.

Pets

Without a doubt, the thought of having to give up a pet can be a deal breaker when discussing and investigating the possibility of moving to assisted living. Thankfully, communities have increasingly recognized this important relationship and in many, animals are fully embraced with open arms. Not only will you find cats and dogs, but some residents will have birds, fish, rabbits, and other small animals. These facilities have reported an increase in the overall health of their residents and some even claim an increase in the residents' projected life spans!

Activities

What did your loved ones enjoy doing before the move? Were they active and involved in the local senior center or did they prefer maintaining a small herb garden on their patio? For some, a robust game of cards or rummikub is enjoyed. Their minds are still sharp and they enjoy the competition. Others may seek more relaxing activities, such as watching television or a movie with friends or reading quietly at home or in the library. Assisted living communities focus

For most of his life, my dad was an avid poker player. Unfortunately, as he aged, he developed macular degeneration and glaucoma. Frustrated, he quit playing with his friends at the assisted living center and fell into a deep depression. He had no other interests, and the staff realized that he was spending too much time alone.

We insisted Dad go with a group of residents to the local senior center for lunch and just to get outside for a drive. Much to his delight, he discovered a group of people who were all in various stages of visual decline playing cards. Several were using very large magnifying glasses to read the cards while one woman was wearing a set of binoculars that looked like reading glasses! They also had several decks of cards with oversized print. Dad realized that he wasn't the only one suffering from vision loss, and there were ways he might be able to continue playing cards.

Dad made his way around the table, introducing himself, and asking if he could try their equipment out. He couldn't have been more excited if he was six years old and it was Christmas morning. By the next day, Dad and I were at the local store for the visually impaired buying binoculars and oversized cards.

The next week, Dad returned to his usual card game and showed everyone his new equipment. Amazingly, several others opened up about having similar problems and expressed gratitude for his sharing. Today, almost everyone at the community is asking him for solutions to their eyesight difficulties. *—Rick*

on providing a variety of activities that will provide social and/or mental stimulation for all residents, regardless of abilities or interest.

One of the most important activities for seniors is sharing a meal. This is the perfect setting for people to come together and interact, sharing stories of their day, remembering past events, and discussing life in general. While mealtime may not be a big deal to those who are younger and active, meals may be the only activity some residents are able to participate in, and they provide a rich source of social stimulation.

Stimulation comes in many forms, and it's important for family and friends to understand that what one resident desires or needs doesn't necessarily suit another resident. For those with dementia—especially Alzheimer's disease—it may be more interesting and pleasurable to interact one-on-one with a caregiver or visitor and talk about the past, relating stories of their childhood, wedding, babies, and pets.

Remember, even if a resident does not participate in an activity, simply being near others and watching or listening will provide a level of stimulation that person would not receive living alone at home.

Health Care

Although the professional and medical qualifications of each assisted living community may vary, they offer similar benefits to their residents. Many have nurses on staff or on-call 24 hours a day, and it is common practice for doctors to contract with communities and visit regularly. Residents may sign up with these doctors, eliminating the need to leave the community for appointments other than those with specialists. In some instances, services such as x-rays, blood work, therapies, and dentistry can be brought directly to the community.

If a resident wants to retain his current doctors, and transportation is provided at the community, he will be able to use the center's bus or town car to get to the appointments and free up the family from that responsibility. This can be a tremendous relief for family members struggling to keep up with their own responsibilities and making sure Mom or Dad attend all their medical appointments.

The community's nurse and care giving staff will work with the resident, his doctor, and the family to create a team and oversee all the resident's health care needs. They will supervise medications, coordinate and follow up on doctor's visits, monitor vitals, and much more. Most communities recognize that monitoring a resident's well-being includes not only the physical health needs but also his mental and emotional state. They will work with the family to ensure that their loved one is as healthy and happy as possible.

Quality Time with Family

In a care giving situation, it can be difficult for all parties involved to recognize the effect circumstances have taken on personal relationships. Roles become reversed when children care for parents. Family members disagree and divide over caregiving responsibilities. Romantic intimacy is lost when one spouse cares for the other. One of the most powerful benefits assisted living can offer is the return and healing of family roles.

Once the primary caregiving responsibilities are handed over to the community and its staff, relationships can return to their previous roles. Instead of spending your time together providing care, quality time can be spent enjoying each other's company.

Types of Residential Eldercare Communities Available

One of the most difficult decisions you will make is when you reach the conclusion that your loved one is unable to remain in his or her own home or live with family, and there needs to be a change in living arrangements. Assisted living becomes the appropriate option when there have usually been numerous emergencies or difficulties in providing suitable care at home and all other options have been exhausted.

When the time has come to begin the process of seeking which type of community would be most appropriate, you may find yourself confused over the numerous choices offered (or at least the terms used to describe them), including assisted living facility, assisted living center, residential care community, continuing care retirement community, private group home, adult care home, assisted living residence, board and care, family care home, memory care community, and Alzheimer's special care unit. Although these are all terms for assisted living facilities, there can be significant differences in size, amenities, and atmosphere. They may also not all provide the same levels or types of care. That is why it's critical to understand what various services different communities provide, what type of care they are licensed for, and the overall atmosphere your senior would experience living there.

Licensing for assisted living facilities is controlled at the state level, and each state has the right to decide how it will refer to these facilities in the state. If you are unsure of the terminology for what you are seeking, visit the websites for your state's department of health services or the Assisted Living Federation of America. Both are great resources for assisted living communities.

The following information will give you a broad understanding of what you can expect if you are exploring assisted living facilities, and it will help you avoid spending unnecessary time investigating the wrong type of community.

Independent Living Communities

There are many communities that encourage and allow fully independent people to move in even though they are licensed for assisted living. To be a good fit in an independent living community, your senior would need little or no assistance with activities of daily living. Your loved one could go into independent living and have a few minor services brought in to assist him or her until enough care is needed to qualify for assisted living.

A perfect example would be a married couple where the wife is healthy, outgoing, and active, but the husband has early stages of Parkinson's disease. Although the husband is social and enjoys living at home, his wife is not comfortable leaving him alone in the afternoon while she enjoys time with her friends. What if he fell or needed something while she was gone? Or perhaps it's becoming too difficult for her to assist him with showering. A good choice would be a community offering both independent and assisted living. They would have their own apartment in the independent section, and some basic services could be provided privately in their residence. The wife could rest assured that her husband could receive any care services needed, and they could still enjoy an active lifestyle using the community's amenities such as the restaurant/bar, swimming pool, and theater.

Assisted Living Communities

There are usually specific needs that indicate a person requires assisted living rather than independent living. Some of these indicators might include but not be limited to: medication management, regular monitoring for medical conditions, or incontinence management.

Assisted living provides supervision or assistance with activities of daily living (ADL); coordination of services by outside health care providers; and the monitoring of resident activities to help to ensure the resident's health, safety, and well-being. Assistance may include the administration or supervision of medication or personal care services such as assistance with showering or toileting provided by trained staff. The goal is to provide care but also to help the resident remain as independent as possible.

Any community you are considering should conduct its own assessment of your loved one to determine what services will be required and that your senior is an appropriate fit for its facility. (See Chapter 9 to learn more about specific considerations relevant to seeking assisted living.)

Memory/Dementia Care Communities

Memory or dementia care is for those who have been diagnosed with Alzheimer's disease or other related dementias. It is for people who are no longer oriented, tend to wander, or present a danger to themselves or to others.

This level of care is very specific, and you will find staff that are trained in dementia care tactics such as distraction and redirection. These communities provide care in a safe, loving environment. While residents can move around on their own within the facility, the main doors to the outside remain locked. A code is required to enter and exit the community to ensure no resident will accidentally find a way out and possibly become lost or injured. Communities usually feature a small private room or a larger shared room. Most feature common areas for the residents to mingle and engage in appropriate activities and may also have secured outdoor courtyards so residents can enjoy being outside in the fresh air.

Continuing Care Retirement Communities

This type of community offers independent living, assisted living, and often memory/dementia care or skilled nursing located on one campus, and residents can move between different levels of care without ever leaving that particular community.

If considering a continuing care retirement community (CCRC), it is important to understand that some of these communities require a large buy-in or entrance fee before moving in—often in the hundreds of thousands of dollars or more! In addition, residents will continue to pay monthly rent and other charges. The buy-in fee is intended to prepay for care and provide the community with operating capital. Potential occupants must look at these communities as an investment, consult with trusted advisors such as an attorney or financial planner, and understand the contract thoroughly before committing.

A common misconception about CCRCs is that a person needs to buy-in in order to live at the community. This is not necessarily true. Many communities will also offer a month-to-month lease with slightly higher monthly fees.

If you are interested in a CCRC for your senior and are considering a buy-in, take a realistic look at your loved one's situation before committing such a large sum of money. For instance, if he is ninety years old, suffers from mid- to late-stage Parkinson's disease, and has been declining over the past year or two, it might not be in his best financial interest to buy-in and give the community a large amount of money up front when he might pass away in the next year or two. A large percentage of that money may not be refundable and will never be put to the use intended.

Skilled Nursing Communities

Skilled nursing facilities, also referred to as nursing homes, offer long- and short-term care for those who suffer from serious or chronic health issues that are too complicated to tend to at home or in an assisted living community.

This type of community provides custodial and skilled nursing care around the clock. Some of the services it can offer that an assisted living community might not include the following:

- postoperative or open wound care

- monitoring intravenous medications

- treatment for an infectious condition

- immediate treatment after a stroke, heart attack, or accident

- late-stage dementia care

They are also capable of providing assistance with activities of daily living such as bathing, dressing, and personal hygiene.

Respite Care Communities

Respite care provides short-term, temporary relief to those who are caring for loved ones who might otherwise require permanent placement in a facility outside the home. With respite care, your loved one can go to a community and receive care for a short time while you or the caregiver take a vacation, attend to health issues of their own, or simply recharge. Respite may also be provided to those who are incapacitated because of an accident or illness and who need assistance during recovery. It is not intended for long-term stays. Normal periods of respite might be a few days to a few weeks.

It is important to note that not all assisted living communities provide respite care.

Understanding Levels of Care and Licensing

Every assisted living facility must be licensed by the state in which it operates, and there are three levels of licensing for different types of care. It is extremely important that you understand what level of care the community is licensed for and the services it can legally provide.

Supervisory Care

Supervisory care is general supervision for those residents who are more independent and highly functioning. Caregivers simply provide a daily awareness of your loved one's ability to function and what his or her needs may be. Limitations include the following:

- There is no hands-on assistance.

- Residents must be able to self-administer medications.

- Caregivers are only allowed to intervene during a crisis, such as assisting after a fall or conducting the Heimlich maneuver if a resident is choking.

Supervisory care is minimum assistance. Residents would need to be able to perform functions, such as the following:

- being able to recognize and respond in an emergency with little to no assistance

- walking/transferring independently with no or infrequent falls

- having no need for hands-on assistance to perform activities of daily living

- being continent of bowel and bladder or being able to manage incontinence themselves

- bathing independently

- being oriented to time, place, and self

- having little memory impairment

- being able to understand the consequences of their actions

Personal Care

Personal care is the next level up from supervisory care. Caregivers are allowed to perform hands-on assistance with activities of daily living such as bathing, dressing, grooming, and mobility. The resident must be able to make basic care decisions, summon assistance, express his or her needs, and recognize danger.

Some needs a resident in a personal care licensed facility might have would include the following:

- assistance recognizing and responding in an emergency

- assistance with transfers and mobility

- medication management, but he or she is still able to self-administer medications

- verbal cues and reminders to perform activities of daily living

- assistance with incontinence management

- assistance with showering or bathing

- encouragement to participate in activities or to socialize

- help with orientation

Directed Care

This is the highest level of care for licensing, and it is given to residents who are unable to make basic care decisions, recognize danger, summon assistance, or express their needs. The caregivers will need to provide direction or perform ADL for the resident, and they are allowed to administer medications or treatments.

In addition to requiring the types of services provided under a personal care license, residents may also need the following:

- assistance in recognizing or responding to an emergency

- medication adjustments and behavior management

* * * * *

When exploring communities, be sure to ask them what level they are licensed for. You can also visit your state's department of health services and look for its database of licensed communities. This will provide the licensing information as well.

Deciding Between a Large Assisted Living Center or a Smaller Assisted Living Group Home

There are two distinct size differences between all communities. If they have more than 11 residents, then they are considered an assisted living center. If they have 10 or fewer residents, then they are considered an assisted living group home. Remember that these terms may be different in your state. Making the decision on whether you should look at a large center or a group home can be confusing. There are important considerations that can help make the decision very clear.

Large Assisted Living Center

In a large assisted living center, residents typically live in their own apartments, but come together for communal meals, socialization, and activities.

Here are some common characteristics of large assisted living centers.

- Residents pay a base rate for the apartment and then pay for care services in addition to the base rate. Utilities (except for phone), maintenance, housekeeping, a certain number of meals, and transportation are included in the base rate.

- Care is provided on a scheduled basis.

- Social, cultural, educational, fitness, and recreational programs are offered.

- There is 24-hour on-site staff.

- Community features and amenities may include, but are not limited to resort-style dining, multiple restaurants, theaters, libraries, chapels with multidenominational services, fitness centers, swimming pools and/or spas, and parking.

Smaller Private Group Homes

Smaller private group homes are more intimate, much like a family environment. Residents either have a private room or share a room. Some homes may offer private bathrooms, but many residents share common bathrooms. Residents are encouraged to consider the entire home their own. They are welcome to have company and use the common areas to entertain or to have guests in their room. In most instances, all residents will come together at mealtime, unless there is a reason for someone to eat in their room.

Caregivers are on-site 24 hours a day. Also, the same caregivers are often at the home daily.

Some of the more common characteristics of these homes may include, but are not limited to, the following things.

- The majority of group homes set a flat rate that includes room, care services, all meals and snacks, housekeeping, and laundry—everything except for certain personal costs like copayments on medications or doctors' appointments, incontinence supplies, private phone, and visits to the beautician.

- Caregivers are always aware of the residents and can often anticipate and meet their requirements before the residents ask or show a need.

- Community features and amenities may include, but are not limited to, home-cooked meals with menus tailored toward specific diets for conditions like diabetes and allergies or personal preferences and group and individual activities such as music, card games, board games, and movies.

* * * * *

As you can see, there are many choices available to you to provide qualified care for your loved one. The issue of who provides that care and where it occurs is a private matter that only you, your loved one, and the family can decide. However, when making these decisions, remember to address not only the health-related needs but also the social, emotional, cultural, intellectual, and spiritual well-being of both the caregiver and the care recipient. When care is taken to identify the most qualified caregiver and the most appropriate living arrangement, the likelihood of successfully meeting physical, mental, and spiritual needs in a qualified and loving manner is greatly increased.

████████████ CAREGIVER SURVIVAL TIP ████████████

There is no possible way to accurately predict how a loved one will age and what challenges your senior may face over the course of his or her journey. As a caregiver, you need to remember that providing care needs to be flexible. What is appropriate today may change drastically tomorrow, and you may need help at some point in time. How can you successfully provide care while adjusting each time a change occurs?

Accept that as needs change, you may require other sources of assistance to ensure your loved one is cared for appropriately.

Educate yourself on the resources available before you need them.

Plan ahead and know who you will turn to when that time comes.

Understand that despite individual preferences and efforts, your options may be limited. You may have to make choices that others don't always agree with, but you are putting the care needs ahead of personal opinions or desires and doing what is necessary.

CHAPTER 6

Paying for Your Loved One's Care

Despite recognizing that you need help in providing care for a loved one and your good intentions in seeking that assistance, the costs for care can be a significant deterrent. One of the biggest challenges seniors and families face today when deciding on eldercare options is how to pay for it. Many mistakenly believe that Medicare or Medicaid will provide the funds for their long-term care should they ever need it. In fact, these two programs pay for rehabilitative or curative care, not custodial care.

Many of our seniors lived their lives believing that they would "self-insure" and save enough money to be able to handle any costs associated with their golden years. However, they may have significantly underestimated what their needs might be or how much they would cost. The recent recession caused a great upheaval for many families and individuals who may have felt they had enough savings or investments to cover any form of assistance required. Retirement accounts and investments were hit hard and now those accounts may be significantly smaller.

There are also those elders who have lived with the belief that if they ever needed significant care or had to leave their own home, they would move in with their children. The common scenario of the stay-at-home mom who tended to all family needs, such as taking care of the children or aging relatives, has now been replaced by two-income families struggling just to make ends meet or single parent households with no extra time or energy to devote to providing care for a declining loved one.

Determining how to pay for your senior's care may cause a few grey hairs, but with a thorough understanding of eldercare options available, accurate pricing for those choices, knowledge of financial resources to help pay for care, and careful fiscal planning, even those with limited budgets can expect to be able to put some form of care in place.

UNDERSTANDING AVERAGE COSTS OF CARE

At some point in time, it's likely that you will have to make decisions for your loved one, like when in-home assistance is needed for your loved one or when living at home is no longer an option. Realistically, while you might have an idea of what you would prefer as far as the type of care and location, the actual costs may affect those decisions.

The average costs for long-term care vary greatly depending on the type of care needed and the geographical area—in urban areas, you can expect that costs will be higher than those in nonurban areas. How do you even begin to understand what the bottom line will be when beginning the search for caregiving assistance? One reliable source would be Genworth, a leader in the long-term care industry, whose *2014 Cost of Care Survey* noted the following median costs for various types of care nationwide.

- **Homemaker services–$19 per hour.** This service is for those who wish to live in their own homes, or to return to their homes, but need assistance with tasks such as cooking, cleaning, or running errands that do not require touching of the care recipient.

- **Home health aide services–$20 per hour.** This service provides assistance, such as help with toileting or showering, to those who live in their own homes instead of residential care facilities or nursing homes. Often, this care is more extensive than family or friends have the time or resources to provide.

- **Adult day health care–$65 per day.** This service is a planned program that provides socialization, supervision, and structured activities for individual needs in a safe, supportive, and cheerful environment. These centers can offer a much-needed break to caregivers.

- **Assisted living facility–$3,500 per month.** These facilities are long-term or permanent living arrangements that provide a wide variety of personal care and health services for people who may need assistance with activities of daily living (ADL). It is an intermediate solution for people who cannot remain at home but are not ready for a nursing home.

- **Nursing home care–$212 (semiprivate room) to $240 (private room) per day.** These facilities are for seniors who are unable to care for themselves, typically suffering from severe or debilitating illnesses—either physical or mental—and requiring 24-hour monitoring and medical care.

Please note that the names for the various types of communities or facilities can be different across the nation and are often interchangeable. Some may refer to them as assisted living facilities, while others may call them continuing care communities; a private group home may be known as a residential care home; and a memory care facility might be referred to as a nursing home. It is important to understand the terms your state uses when identifying where your loved one would be an appropriate fit. A good way to do this is to visit your state's department of health and human services and research its listings for communities.

When our dad had a stroke, the hospital sent him to a skilled nursing center that cost $294 a day. That's over $8,000 a month. The damage from the stroke was significant, and he wasn't going to be able to return home and live on his own. We didn't know how we were going to be able to afford it if he remained at the center indefinitely. With some careful research, we found an assisted living community that was licensed at a level that could provide the care he needed with some additional services brought in by a home health agency. The total cost for this arrangement was a little over $4,500. It's still terribly expensive, but knowing what's available and how much it will cost makes a difference. Nobody should just assume that the first answer is the best. We're hoping that, over time, he'll recover enough that he'll be able to go home, with the home health agency coming to his house, and we'll save even more money. —*Phillip*

DETERMINING NEEDS AND BUDGETING FOR COSTS OF CARE

Part of the problem in budgeting for health care needs is that they are often fluid, making it difficult to accurately predict the cost of care over an extended period of time. As our loved one ages, it is likely that her physical and mental health will worsen to some degree, but every senior's journey is unique. It's quite possible that at one point in time she may need significant help, especially if she is recovering from an acute condition like a stroke or heart attack. Of course, as she improves, her needs decrease. But if your loved one requires care because of a chronic condition such as Alzheimer's disease, or if she is fragile because of significant age, then her needs may continue indefinitely and increase over time. In short, the greater the amount of care, the greater the cost.

It's no wonder that making the decision on choosing care services or other living arrangements for your loved one can be a complicated and emotional task. There are three basic steps that can help you begin the process and make it easier.

1. **Determine what the senior's needs are.** As discussed in Chapter 3, identifying and understanding your loved one's needs are the first critical steps in knowing which options to begin exploring. If your mom only needs companionship, then there is no reason to research skilled nursing facilities. If she needs assistance with toileting and medication management, then homemaker services cannot offer the proper level of support.

2. **Identify what services are available to meet those needs and how much they cost.** Depending on where you live, the type of services available may vary from other locations. Research eldercare resources within a reasonable distance from your location and start requesting information on what services they provide and their rates. Reach out to local providers, such as your loved one's health care team, pharmacist, or senior center, to find out about which local agencies they refer, and ask for feedback to assist you in the decision-making process. Another easy source for reviewing the current cost of care and to project future costs in your area is the Genworth Cost of Care Survey—April 2014 (www.genworth.com/corporate/about-genworth/industry -expertise/cost-of-care.html).

3. **Decide how services will be paid.** Once you have actual figures for budgeting, examine any sources available to help pay for care. It may be wise to enlist the aid of a financial advisor to determine how best to use those sources. A list of possible methods to pay for care will follow later in this chapter.

When defining the monthly budget for care, many people correctly estimate the service fees, but fail to identify those smaller recurring costs that could potentially create havoc with their financial planning. The last thing you want to do is to begin services or move your loved one, only to learn later on that you failed to include hidden or unexpected expenses in your budget, which is now stressed or broken. Remember, it is better to overestimate the costs than to underestimate them and have to make changes that may be disruptive to the health and well-being of your loved one. Some items your senior may want or need regularly that should be calculated into the expenses include the following:

- prescriptions
- medical/dental copays
- incontinence supplies (adult diapers, wipes, gloves, etc.)
- assistive devices like walkers, wheelchairs, adjustable beds, or grab bars
- private transportation costs (transportation provided by professional service providers like taxis or buses if family or friends cannot meet the needs)
- entertainment expenses for outings
- groceries
- beauty expenses such as haircuts, manicures, and so on
- pet expenses
- home modifications

IDENTIFYING WAYS TO PAY FOR CARE

It isn't surprising if one of your major concerns relative to providing care is how much it will cost and how you will pay for it. Your first reaction to the initial budget might be shock and then fear. Don't panic—the ability to pay will probably have to come from several different sources grouped together to cover the full cost. Be

Boy did I make some big mistakes when helping my mother create a budget for her future long-term care. She was moving from Minnesota to Colorado so that we could live closer together, and I could help with her care if needed. Even with Parkinson's disease, Mom was independent enough to live on her own, and we purchased a small town home within a few miles of where my husband and I live.

To budget for her new mortgage and prepare for whatever might happen with her health needs down the road, we talked to a few in-home care agencies to get pricing so we wouldn't be caught off guard. The problem is that we didn't take into consideration what it might cost if the disease got worse and she needed some significant changes to her home or other areas of her life. Unfortunately, over the past few months, Mom has significantly declined and can't drive any longer. The doctor has told us that she will need a wheelchair in the foreseeable future. All of this means expensive modifications to her home to make it wheelchair accessible, added transportation service costs, as well as hiring the caregiving agency we had budgeted for. These two expenses alone will make it far too expensive for her to live in this town home any longer. *–Felicia*

reassured that while you may have to pay out of pocket for one expense, another may be covered through insurance, volunteers, or government benefits.

There is one trap that too many families fall into—offsetting the costs with their own savings, home equity, and retirement accounts to help their loved one. It's easy to jump to the conclusion that the only way to pay is through private funds, but that's not always the case. You may unnecessarily spend down your own money and jeopardize your future when there might have been other available resources that could have reduced the amount of money coming out of your

My parents were killed in a car accident when I was four years old. I am an only child and the only other close relative I had was my mother's sister, Aunt Mary. Even though Aunt Mary was a widow, she took me in and raised me as her own. It has always been her desire to pass peacefully in her own home and, after what she did for me, I intended to honor that wish. As she has aged, I have done my best to care for her.

I was promoted two years ago, my hours have drastically increased, and it's been necessary to travel for my job. Since I'm not available to help Aunt Mary or visit as much as I use to, I've hired a home care agency to cover those times when I'm unavailable. I've been paying for this cost and felt it was the least I could do. I know that Aunt Mary's monthly income would not cover the costs. To date, I have nearly exhausted my savings, and I was worried I would have to withdraw from my retirement account.

Thankfully, I was discussing this possibility with my human resources department when they asked me if either Aunt Mary or her late husband had been a veteran. Uncle Saul was, and much to my surprise and delight, Aunt Mary was entitled to a pension benefit through the VA as his surviving spouse. This benefit will pay over a $1,000 a month towards the costs of the caregivers. Also, the HR department suggested I contact Duet, a nonprofit agency here in Phoenix that uses volunteers to partner with families and individuals to assist with eldercare.

Not only will I be able to apply the money from the VA to her professional care, but she now has a companion who comes on a regular basis from Duet.

I wish I had discussed my situation when I first realized I would need help in caring for Aunt Mary. I could have saved thousands of dollars of my own money and still provided for her. I just didn't realize there were other sources available to help. —*Tess* pockets. Take time to carefully evaluate any form of income coming to your senior or resources available before you spend your own money.

As you will see in the following sections, there are options other than risking your own financial future to pay for care. There are four possible categories you can draw upon to fund you elder's care. Within these four categories, there are a number of possibilities available from financial assistance to help with other specific needs such as reduced prescriptions or free support groups. Here is a key sampling of those choices.

Personal Property

Often, utilizing personal property is the most immediate means for paying for care. These assets can be tangible or intangible possessions. Tangible resources include anything you can touch and move such as jewelry, cars, and furniture. They can easily be liquidated into funds, while intangible possessions might take much longer and more effort. Intangible materials include whatever you can't take hold of and where your ownership is conveyed through a piece of paper like insurance policies, stocks, or home equity. Some of the most common methods for paying for assisted living care through personal property are listed in the following sections.

Private Funds

Private funds can come from a variety of sources such as savings, personal investments like 401K plans or IRAs, or other assets that people have accumulated. When identifying what money is available, start with the obvious—social security, pension, and other forms of monthly income. Next, move on to savings and retirement accounts. When considering withdrawing monies from investments and retirement accounts, it is advisable to consult with your accountant or financial planner first to discuss penalties, tax liabilities, or whether there may be other means available that you haven't considered before depleting private funds.

Home Equity

The equity in your elder's home may be a valuable source to pay for care. Much will depend on the amount of equity available and how much and for how long care will be required. If the home is not paid in full, if there are other large monthly expenses, or if care will exceed the available loan amount over time, this may not be the best solution. The downside to obtaining a conventional home equity loan would be that your elder is required to pay it back with interest, which may strain his or her budget.

Reverse Mortgage

Another way in which older adults can tap in to the equity of their home is through a reverse mortgage. One of the biggest differences between a reverse mortgage and a home equity loan is that with a home equity loan, your seniors may need to show proof of an adequate income level in order to make repayments. With a reverse mortgage, the homeowners can convert their equity into cash with no repayment required until they die, move out, or sell their home. A reverse mortgage gives them access to tax-free cash—only withdrawing money as they need it.

To apply for a reverse mortgage, your senior must meet the following qualifications.

- The applicant must be at least 62 years of age.
- The applicant must occupy the home as the principal residence.
- The applicant must own the home outright or have a minimal balance that could be paid off with proceeds from the loan.

- The home must be a single-family dwelling or a two- to four-unit property that the senior owns and occupies.

Renting or Selling the Home

While your senior's home may be his or her biggest asset, and there may be great emotional attachment, sometimes circumstances dictate the need for a new plan regarding ownership. If it becomes apparent that your loved one would be better off moving in with you or to a care community, then perhaps the best solution is to rent the home or sell it outright.

Rick Wandrych, Real Estate Broker, Senior Real Estate Specialist, and Certified Probate Real Estate Specialist, notes the pros and cons to both options.

Benefits to Renting

- It provides monthly income that will help offset any assisted living expenses.
- The home remains in the family estate.
- There is possible continued appreciation.
- Your loved one can move back home if he or she improves.

Downside to Renting

- It requires a landlord or a property management company.
- It requires the senior to continue paying taxes, mortgages, upkeep, or any other expenses related to homeownership.

Benefits to Selling

- The senior receives a lump sum of money.
- The proceeds can be reinvested, and the gains can be used to offset the costs of assisted living.

My ninety-year-old mother lives off her monthly social security. It's not much, but she has managed over the years. Fortunately, her home is paid in full. During the last six months, Mom had some recurring health issues that resulted in surgery and several stays in the hospital. She needed a caregiver to stay with her during those recoveries. Mom was reluctant to accept help because she couldn't afford to and didn't want her children paying for it.

Because this condition will continue to be an issue for her off and on, I insisted that we talk with a financial advisor who suggested a reverse mortgage to cover the costs. It's worked out very well, and she will only draw money from the account when she needs the care. Because there are no payments until she passes away or has to move from her home to a care community, she doesn't feel the effects of the price of her care. —*Aubrey*

- There are no additional expenses related to homeownership.
- The senior is no longer exposed to real estate market fluctuations.

Downside to Selling

- Your loved one will not be able to move back home if he or she improves.

Insurance Coverage

One of the biggest misconceptions that families or seniors have with regard to paying for eldercare is that most forms of insurance will cover all long-term care expenses. While it's likely that your loved one's health, long-term care, or Medicare coverage will offset specific costs, it's also likely your senior will have to mix and match benefits to pay for the majority of or all related expenditures. It's wise to thoroughly read the benefits section of his or her policies before assuming protection. In the following sections, Maryglenn Boals, founder of MgBoals and Associates, a long-term care planning firm in Phoenix, Arizona, explains the four common forms of insurance that may help your elder afford assisted living solutions.

Life Insurance Conversion

Converting life insurance to cash is one way of securing a large amount of money to pay for eldercare expenses. However, this option is not available with term life insurance, as it has no cash value. Also known as a life settlement, it involves the sale of an insurance policy by the policyholder to a third party in exchange for a defined amount of long-term care services while preserving a death benefit. Your loved one would sell the life insurance policy for an agreed-upon dollar value, and the buyer takes over the monthly premium payments and then collects the death benefits when the policyholder dies. The advantages include the following:

- available funds for long-term care

- no more premiums

- funds to pay off other debt

The major disadvantage to this option is that when your senior dies, the family will not receive the death benefit from the life insurance. The third party that purchased the policy is the new beneficiary.

Long-Term Care Insurance

This is an important form of insurance that will provide coverage where health insurance ends. Long-term care (LTC) refers to when your loved one's condition progresses to the point where constant supervision or assistance with activities of daily living like bathing, toileting, and dressing is required. LTC insurance will provide funds to help cover these expenses. If your loved one qualifies, payments can be made to care providers in the home, for respite stays or adult day care, or for assisted living facilities and skilled nursing facilities.

Medicare

Medicare covers only medically necessary care such as doctor visits, drugs, hospital stays, and short-term services for conditions that will improve, like physical therapy to help you regain your function after a fall or a stroke. Medicare does not pay for long-term care services, personal care with activities of daily living, or custodial care. Medicare will pay for short-term stays in a skilled nursing facility, for hospice care, and home health care. To qualify, your loved one would need to have had a recent hospital stay of at least three days; need to be admitted to a Medicare certified nursing home within thirty days of the prior hospital stay; and need skilled care such as skilled nursing services, physical therapy, or other types of therapy.

Other Health Insurance

Most private health insurances or employer HMOs follow the same general rules as Medicare with regard to paying for long-term care services. The majority of private insurance policies do not cover personal or custodial care. If they do cover these care services, it is typically only for skilled, short-term, medically necessary care.

- Home care coverage is limited to medically necessary skilled care.

- Admittance to and coverage for a skilled nursing facility must follow a recent hospital stay for the same condition or a related one. Your loved one's stay in skilled nursing is limited to one hundred days for payment through health insurance.

- Medicare Supplemental Insurance (Medigap) are private policies that will fill in some of the gaps in Medicare coverage, such as covering Medicare copayments and deductibles. It is not intended to meet long-term care needs.

While private policies do not cover long-term care expenses, they can free up funds by covering other costs. This may make a difference in the ability to budget for eldercare.

Government Programs

The budgets of many seniors and their families are stretched to the breaking point when forced to pay for eldercare expenses. Fortunately, there are several government programs that can provide assistance in covering these costs. Here are some suggestions to investigate to see if your loved one might qualify for assistance.

Medicaid

Medicaid Long-Term Care is a jointly funded, state and federal insurance program for low-income seniors and disabled individuals. It provides medical care and support services. If your loved one is financially and medically qualified, Medicaid will pay nearly all the long-term care costs.

Medicaid Waivers are Medicaid programs in specific states that provide care and support to individuals outside of nursing homes— usually at home, in assisted living facilities, or in adult day care environments. These waivers are not entitlements, and have enrollment caps and often have waiting lists.

Cash and Counseling (also known as Participant/Consumer or Self-Directed Program) is a specific type of Medicaid Waiver program available in many states. Your senior receives funds for care and the flexibility to select his or her own care providers, including family members in some instances. Payments can be paid directly to you. Contact your Medicaid office to see if your state qualifies.

Veteran's Benefits

Seniors who are also veterans may be eligible for a wide variety of benefits, including disability compensation, pension, insurance, health care, long-term care, and burial. Certain elderly veterans can receive additional monetary compensation if they are eligible for or receiving a VA Pension benefit.

The VA Improved Pension (also known as the Aid and Attendance Benefit) provides an increased monthly pension if your loved one requires help performing activities of daily living, is bedridden, resides in a nursing home, or has severely limited eyesight. The Improved Pension may be granted to a veteran or a surviving spouse.

The Housebound benefit is another increased monthly pension paid to seniors if they are confined to their immediate premises because of a permanent disability.

There are individuals or organizations that can assist individuals/ families in the application process and claim to speed up the process by ensuring everything is complete before submission. You can search the Internet for assistance with the VA Aid and Attendance Pension. The following organizations would be a good place to start for guidance.

- www.veteranaid.org
- www.veteransaidbenefit.org

Area Agencies on Aging

Area Agencies on Aging (AAAs) are local aging programs that provide information and services on a range of assistance for older adults and those who care for them. Your local agency can help you access critical information including the following:

- available services in your area
- mobility assistance programs, meal plans, and housing
- assistance in gaining access to services
- individual counseling, support groups, and caregiver training
- respite care
- supplemental services on a limited basis

I've been my dad's primary caregiver for the past three years. He still lives on his own but requires assistance getting going every morning—showering, cooking breakfast, taking his meds—and then again at night getting ready for bed. Frankly, I'm worn out and would like my time and freedom back. Dad has refused to move to a small assisted living facility near my home because he doesn't want to spend the money. I'd be happy to help out financially, but I can't carry the full cost.

Recently, I attended a seminar on the VA Aid and Attendance Benefit and found out that Dad was eligible for almost $1,800 a month to use towards the cost of the facility. Since the monthly rate is just a little over $3,000, this benefit will pay more than half. Although he still doesn't want anyone to have to spend any money on the facility, he has agreed to move because he doesn't want to lose out on any benefit he earned fighting for our country. I am so grateful for this benefit. *–Aaron*

Some agencies will even assist you in preparing applications and documentation.

Social Security
Social Security is a federal program providing retirement income to seniors or the permanently disabled. Seniors commonly use it as a source to cover long-term care expenses. An individual must have paid social security taxes while employed in order to qualify.

Payments are made directly to the individual and can be applied in any manner needed, such as home care or residential care. Each person receives a sum calculated on the amount and number of years paid into the system along with the age at which he or she chose to receive benefits.

Supplemental Security Income (SSI) helps financially needy seniors with extremely limited income and assets, filling the gap to bring their income up to a predetermined level. The benefit amount is dependent on their current income. Unlike Social Security benefits, it is not based on an individual's prior work. These funds can also be applied in any way chosen to pay for eldercare expenses.

Private Assistance

While there may be limited resources that will assist with direct funding for long-term care, other resources are available that can provide financial relief in other areas and free up money for the actual care itself. Here are two potential resources that may have been overlooked and could save you money to use on other needs.

Prescription Drug Assistance

There are multiple ways that you can save money on prescriptions. For example, NeedyMeds.org is a nonprofit organization offering a free card that helps families obtain prescription drugs at the lowest possible cost. Also, patient assistance programs are run by nearly all the major pharmaceutical companies and offer assistance to low-income individuals by providing reduced cost or free medicines. In addition, using mail-order or online pharmacies can provide savings over purchasing your medication directly from a retail pharmacy.

Nonprofit and Foundation Assistance

Many organizations are disease specific, but offer resources for those suffering from specific conditions. If your loved one has a condition that is contributing to a need for care, research that disorder, and you may find that there is a nonprofit or foundation geared toward helping individuals find resources that could benefit them financially, emotionally, or physically, such as free support groups, affordable respite care, or discounted medical equipment.

CAREGIVER SURVIVAL TIP

The number of programs, benefits, and resources available can be vast and difficult to navigate on your own. Payingforseniorcare .com is a website maintained by the American Elder Care Research Organization. Its Eldercare Financial Resource Locator Tool is designed to help families and caregivers locate information about long-term care resources and to find public and private programs available to assist in covering the cost of such care.

CHAPTER 7

Having the Difficult Discussions

There are certain discussions that are more difficult for family members to have than others. This is especially true when the subject is the physical or mental decline of a loved one. The discussions, which could be one or several, involve what changes may be needed and what that means not only for the individual in question but for the family unit as a whole. Family dynamics can complicate the matter further. Whether it's a single relative, multiple siblings, or other family members monitoring and determining an individual's future, the roles each play can become tense, if not downright combative. Chances are that not everyone involved will see the circumstances the same way or agree with the plan of action discussed as the solution to provide the best care.

Usually within a family, there will be some who won't agree that something needs to change. Most likely, this will be your loved one, although it can be anyone who is in denial, has something to hide, or believes everyone else is wrong.

It takes a great deal of observation, consideration, and planning to have these discussions without causing hurt feelings and family rifts. It may not always work, but if you take time to consider the best manner in which to have them, where to have them, and how to honor everyone's feelings without sacrificing the best interests of your loved one, there is a good chance you will succeed.

BRINGING THE FAMILY TOGETHER

The issues surrounding a loved one who is in decline or has suffered a crisis are difficult and stressful. Bringing a family together to address these issues can be complicated and difficult. Often, adult children or other relatives do not live in the same geographic location, and timing is critical. Perhaps they don't have a good relationship now or never have. Adding in the stress of facing a loved one who may be very resistant to the idea of change, it's easy to see why tempers fly, egos bruise, and feelings get hurt. It can take a great deal of patience and effort to bring everyone together and get everyone on the same page where your elder is concerned. Typically, one person has to take the lead and begin the process.

Usually, those who easily and successfully manage this type of situation have had healthy, respectful relationships with their family in the past. When the relationships aren't so good, coming together as an effective team can be almost impossible. One of the first things to do when faced with the necessity of discussing your loved one's condition and needed solutions is to reach out to those who aren't getting along and mend fences as quickly and effectively as you can. This will help prevent future conversations from turning into a time-wasting game of "Who's to Blame" or an overall complaint session that loses focus on the important matter at hand—your loved one's needs and care. The following steps offer some direction as how to begin the process of uniting the family and creating an atmosphere where you can all work together respectfully and productively.

- Make a list of all family members that have a vested interest in your loved one and would want to participate in her care.

You may have to draw a hard line with some and inform them that they won't be involved if they aren't willing to participate in the caregiving and financial aspects or other means of positive support. This doesn't mean that you won't inform them of important matters or listen to their opinion, it just means they may not have as strong of a say in the decision-making process, if any.

- **Decide how communication will best be handled.** This might be in person, over the phone, text messages, e-mail, or Skype. Remember that people communicate differently, and you may have to use several different methods.

- **Reach out with goodwill.** Make sure family members know they are being contacted because you understand they care and would want to be involved. Let them know you appreciate their advice and help.

- **Acknowledge that everyone has the right to an opinion.** Explain that everyone will have a chance to be heard.

- **Inform them that, if there is disagreement, the services of an unbiased third party may have to be enlisted.** That third party could be a professional mediator.

- **Stress that if someone is not up for participating in the process, she will not be judged.** By the same token, make it clear that she will also not have the right to complain about any outcomes she doesn't agree with.

- **Remind everyone that this is about your loved one and not each other.** This is the time to come together and work on behalf of somebody who needs all of you.

- **Reinforce anything positive about your relationship with all concerned, and thank everyone for being a part of the solution to the situation.**

If you are part of a family that is close and gets along well, then you are lucky! Nonetheless, it still helps to follow some, if not all, of the aforementioned steps to ensure that everyone understands the ground rules for communication and how decisions will be made. Having the family in agreement (as much as possible) makes it easier to discuss what is being noticed, thoughts on how to improve the situation, and resources that need to be considered.

DEVELOPING A STRATEGY FOR YOUR DISCUSSION

Creighton Abrams, the US Army general who commanded military operations in the Vietnam War, once said "When eating an elephant, take one bite at a time." This can easily apply to handling a difficult conversation or an overwhelming situation—break it down into smaller pieces and tackle each one separately.

After you've mended fences when necessary, and are ready to begin your discussion, it's best to have a strategy in place to manage the multiple personalities, interests, and desires. It's also important to recognize personal boundaries. One family member may be fully engaged as a caregiver and handling it well, while another may feel that he can only contribute financially because he was never emotionally close to the senior. Keep an open mind and do not judge anyone by the boundaries he sets. By being gracious and listening, you will make everyone feel respected and safe to speak his mind.

Whether to include your loved one in the early discussions may be unclear at first. There can be some cases where involving your senior would not be advisable. Here are a few guidelines as to if or when to include him.

- If there is serious discord among family members, especially among siblings, attempt to resolve some of these issues first, and find common ground regarding your loved one before involving him. It can be disturbing for a parent to

Earlier this year, my mother had several seizures and fell down the front steps during the most recent attack. She didn't break any bones, but was bruised and cut badly. It really shook me up. Because we are scattered all over the country, I'm the family member who checks in on her regularly. It's been difficult getting everyone to understand my concerns. My brother has been very vocal about the fact that he talks to her every week, and she seems fine to him.

We are going to be together this Thanksgiving for the first time in six years. I'm asking that all the siblings meet after the holiday and discuss what we may have noticed while visiting with her and if we can do anything to help her in her own home or if she should move to a community.

The biggest issue is that my oldest brother (who has power of attorney for Mom) and I had a falling out a few years ago, and now anything I bring up will result in him automatically taking the other stance. It's difficult to go against him, as most of my siblings look up to him and will follow his lead. I've realized that I need to swallow my pride and reach out to him to develop a rapport so that we can realistically discuss Mom. I've written him a heartfelt letter and apologized for my part in our argument. I also stressed that we need to do anything we can to take care of Mom, and that includes working together.

To my surprise, he responded quite well and we've had our first sincere, in-depth conversation since the fight. He's working with me by talking to Mom's medical team and creating a profile of her condition and what we can expect in the future. Once we have this, we will approach the other kids and develop a strategy on how to talk with Mom while we are all there and then decide who will be responsible for what.

I'm so grateful that I reached out and that my brother responded the way he did. *–Lisa* see his children fighting, and even worse if they are fighting because of him.

- Include your loved one from the start if he has recognized the need for care and initiated conversations with you or other family members about the challenges involved.

- If anything that needs to be discussed would be embarrassing or hurtful to your loved one, and having him there will inhibit honest and open conversation, then perhaps his participation should come at a later time. For instance, if your father has not realized he's been having accidents in public and walks around with stains on his pants, you might want to talk in private and discuss a solution. Then you can discuss it with him alone, so that he won't feel ashamed or self-conscious.

- If your senior is resistant to any suggestions that he needs care, and you feel the discussion will be met with anger, resentment, or hostility, it's best to have the initial discussion without him. You can then develop a strategy on how to raise the issue and make sure everyone concerned is on the same page first.

- Finally, if your loved one has dementia, or for some other reason cannot understand or remember what you are discussing, then you need to move forward without him. This can change once some decisions have been made and a plan of action established. If you include your loved one too soon, he may become confused, anxious, or frightened.

Once it's been decided who will be included in the conversation, the following suggestions will be helpful in ensuring that everyone is comfortable and able to speak freely and that the meeting will be productive.

- **Set an agenda and make sure everyone knows what topics will be discussed.** Ask in advance if anyone has a specific matter she would like to talk about and include it. Now is the time to get it all out in the open.

- **Establish ground rules that everyone will have a chance to talk.** All others must listen politely and give the others their time.

- **Recruit one or more members of the discussion to take notes.** Thoughts and ideas can be revisited, if needed.

- **Ask that participants be prepared and have facts to support their ideas.** For instance, if you feel she can't afford to move to a community, but could stay in her own home if she hired a housecleaning service and a landscaper, have pricing available for both options so that you can show financial proof for your suggestion.

- **Remember that there can be more than one solution to a problem, and be willing to compromise.**

- **Agree to disagree.** Insist that participants be courteous and civil toward others.

- **End the meeting by reiterating what was decided, what has to happen before the next meeting, who is in charge of what, and when the next meeting will occur.**

Although these suggestions will help prepare you for the meeting, there are situations where a little private coaching on how to respond or handle specific comments or attitudes can be helpful. The following are common statements that will give you some ideas on how to respond or diffuse resistance:

- **"I don't think Mom needs any care. She seemed fine to me at Christmas."** This is a common attitude, especially when one member is the caregiver and the remaining family doesn't contribute much, if any, to the care of their loved one, particularly if they live in another state. Point out that an individual can often pull it all together for a few hours or days to present a perfect picture to someone he or she has short periods of contact with. A good way to respond to this is, "I don't think you understand what I see daily or what I personally do to help Mom. If you don't recognize or believe what is happening and how hard I'm working at providing care, then I suggest you let Mom come live with you for a while, or you can come home and take care of her for a while. I'm sure you will appreciate my concerns then. Otherwise, I need your support in making these decisions and doing what needs to be done."

- **"I don't understand why we pay for Dad to live in a community. I can move in with him, and he can pay me instead."** There are cases where this could be an ideal answer to a caregiving dilemma, but proceed with caution. Think hard about the reputation of the person moving in. Does the person have a history of responsible behavior? It is not uncommon to see a relative who has had a track record of money problems, is unable to hold a job, or has suffered from drug/alcohol abuse to offer this solution because it is to that person's benefit. They may have great intentions in the beginning, but if he or she loses interest, falls off the wagon, abuses the situation, or fails to provide adequate care, then your loved one may suffer.

   A great way to address this suggestion is to say, "I understand that you want to help Dad and that it would be an ideal arrangement for you, but there would be some requirements for the family to consider you moving in and becoming the primary caregiver. Are you willing to take training classes and become a certified caregiver? Will you sign an employee agreement or will you be an independent contractor? We would want to make sure taxes are being properly paid. If we move forward, I will insist on more than one person having access to Dad's bank and financial records to ensure full transparency. Are you comfortable reporting back to the family? If not, then maybe we need to seek another way to make sure Dad is taken care of."

- **"I don't have time to deal with this. Aunt June is a danger to herself. She needs to move into a care home right now."** Sometimes in a rush to fix a problem, family members will jump to the final solution in what should be a longer journey through multiple options. Taking more time and exhausting each and every option available may make more sense. "I know that you are worried about Aunt June, and I agree that something needs to be done, but I think you're jumping into having her move out of her home too fast. Yes, she isn't taking as good of care of herself or the home as she should, but she's perfectly capable of working with us to figure out what help is needed and then hiring someone. Plus, she loves her home, has friends in the neighborhood, and would miss her senior center. I'd like to give her a chance to bring support into her home, see how it works, and then if or when that doesn't work any longer, we can talk about the possibility of her moving to a community."

One final word of advice: Remember that it is always appropriate and OK to say that you need time to think about what has just been discussed before you answer or agree to anything. Ask for a few hours or a day or two to digest the information and get back to the family on your feelings. Stepping away for a short period of time can bring clarity to the moment and help you make the right choices.

My sister, Paula, and I are ten years apart and didn't spend much time growing up together. She has always lived in the same town as Mom, but as soon as I graduated from high school, I moved two hours away and rarely visited either of them. Because of our age difference, I haven't always felt close to Paula, and frankly, sometimes I think she was jealous of me being the baby in the family.

When Paula first started mentioning she was noticing a physical decline and was concerned about some odd comments from Mom, I immediately became defensive. My sister has always been very dramatic and I thought she was just overexaggerating or even making things up. She would tell me about Mom complaining of horrible side effects from medication or that she was in pain and couldn't move. There were a few times Paula would call in tears because Mom had yelled at her. I would just ignore it and told myself Paula wanted attention and for me to feel guilty that she was the only one taking care of Mom. It's true that I rarely spent much time with Mom, but when I did, I didn't notice anything unusual. I found myself immediately dismissing everything Paula said and often wouldn't even answer the phone when she called.

One day, Paula phoned and said Mom was being transported to the hospital. She was in extreme pain and throwing up. When I got there, Mom was having a complete meltdown and behaving exactly the way Paula described so many times. She was so melodramatic that even the hospital staff was growing impatient with her. I was completely floored by what I was seeing and realized that Mom behaved one way with me and another way with Paula. I felt horrible that I hadn't listened to what my sister had been trying to tell me.

During the week that Mom was hospitalized, Paula and I spent some quality time together discussing the reality of

Mom's health and what help or changes we would need moving forward. Today, we are working together regarding Mom's care. If something happens, Paula and I discuss it respectfully, and both of us offer our opinion and suggestions. Then we approach Mom as a team. What's interesting is that Mom has realized her kids are working together now, and she's behaving differently. She's been more agreeable to allowing others to help her and giving us both the same information about her needs. The hidden blessing to my Mom being hospitalized is that it has brought my sister and me closer together.
—Bill

DOING YOUR HOMEWORK FIRST

One of your most powerful tools for family conversations is to become educated on all topics that might arise. This might include what resources can provide support, what the cost will be, and how you can pay for it. By preparing and knowing how you will address any questions or complaints, you will be better able to handle any fear, anger, or other emotions that may develop.

Earlier in this chapter, you learned how to bring your family together to begin discussing any health concerns related to your loved one. You have met and have come to terms with the idea of either bringing care into the private home or moving your senior to a care community. Now the most difficult discussion(s) of all must happen— speaking with your loved one about your worries, suggestions, and perhaps laying it all out and telling your senior what has to happen whether he or she agrees or not. Your first steps in making this meeting as successful as possible are to gather your facts, determine what resistance to expect, and think ahead about how to address that resistance thoughtfully and knowledgably. Understand that this may be the first of several discussions that may need to take place before your senior is ready to entertain your point of view.

The two biggest obstacles to any change will be your loved one's fears and his or her desire to maintain control. It's difficult for many to understand what our elders have seen or grown up with. Most will tell you that their parents and grandparents took in older relatives and cared for them at home. Those who weren't able to do so had to send them to nursing homes where the philosophy and practices were significantly different than they are today. Your elder may remember people being abandoned by family, drugged until they couldn't function, and sometimes abused. Who can blame them for worrying about this once you point out that they need more help than the family can provide?

You can combat this fear by pulling together as much proof as possible that it will be different before approaching them. Here are some issues that will support you when discussing your concerns and suggestions as to how to solve them.

- **Your loved one needs minimal help with chores around the house.** This is perhaps the easiest need to begin with. Make a list of what you notice each time you visit—items that need repairing, yard work left undone or neglected, disarray or clutter in the home, bad odors or filth, rotten and expired food, or any other signs that your loved one is no longer able meet the normal day-to-day care of his or her home. If necessary, take pictures.

- **Your senior looks disheveled or smells bad, you don't think he or she is eating well or bathing regularly, or perhaps you see signs that your loved one isn't managing medications properly.** Document how often you notice any particular indicator of self-neglect. Speak with your elder's pharmacist or anyone who visits the home about your concerns. Include their comments in your documentation.

- **Your elder has declined to the point that you feel he or she is unsafe alone at home and needs to move.** Keep a record of your concerns and how often problems are occurring. Did Mom fall three times last month? Was Dad admitted to the hospital twice in six months because he mixed up his medications? Have your parents both lost a significant amount of weight because they aren't eating regularly? Did Aunt Phyllis forget about the stove, and a dish towel caught on fire? This is the perfect time to discuss your worries with their medical professionals, neighbors, or any other person who may be able to point out the same observations. Ask if they will support your efforts to move your loved one, if needed.

This documentation will help prevent you from drawing a blank and forgetting what issues you worried about when faced with an argumentative and angry elder.

Next, you need to have as much knowledge and physical evidence about the solutions you are going to suggest as possible. Armed with actual proof rather than guesses or estimates may quickly diffuse your loved one's arguments.

- **Determine what services your loved one needs, and investigate resources.** Identify individuals or agencies that can address those needs and gather information to present. Being able to show your senior a website or a brochure will indicate that you are serious and have done your homework.

- **Get estimates in writing whenever possible.** If you are considering bringing anyone into the home to provide services, like a housecleaner, companion, or home care aide, ask for a formal written estimate. If you can't get a formal estimate, take detailed notes and be able to present quotes to your loved one so there will be no question as to how much it will cost.

- **Discuss details with family members if you are suggesting your senior move in with relatives.** If moving in with family is a possibility, discuss how that will be handled. For example, be able to explain that Mom's two young grandsons are eager to get a bunk bed and share a room so that Grandma can live with them or that her beloved Shih Tzu is welcome and she won't have to give up her pet. The worst thing that can happen is to begin a conversation like this and have your senior discover that it wasn't well thought out or that someone in the household isn't in agreement with the proposed plan.

- **Visit care communities and take pictures, collect information packages, and narrow the options.** If moving in with family isn't an option and the only other solution is that your senior move to a care community, it's imperative that you spend time investigating the possibilities and selecting the best candidates before speaking with your loved one. At this point in time, you may want to enlist the services of an assisted living referral agent who can help you understand the level of care needed, the type of community that would be the best fit, and which communities could best provide those requirements. Then you can do the following:

  ☐ Call and schedule tours with selected communities.

  ☐ Openly and honestly discuss your loved one's needs with the staff member conducting the tour.

  ☐ Take pictures of the community, the grounds, and the apartments or rooms you are shown.

  ☐ Discuss costs and ask for a pricing sheet for base rates and any other expenses related to providing services or care.

  ☐ Ask for an information package to take with you.

Every time I mentioned to my folks that I thought they needed help around the house, they would wave their hands at me. "We don't know what you're so worried about. We're fine." I'd look around and see the home in a mess and know for a fact that they hadn't eaten a home cooked meal all week. I was sure they could really benefit from someone coming in and helping them with just some basic things like cleaning up, laundry, and cooking a bunch of meals to freeze and just pop in the microwave. The problem was that whenever I'd try to bring the subject up, they'd say they couldn't afford it. I know what their monthly retirement income is and what their expenses are—they can afford it.

I finally decided to go out on my own and interview an agency in our town that provides caregivers to do these basic household services. We discussed in detail what I would like done, who would come to the home, how often, and the pricing. The agency gave me a formal estimate and some information on what my parents could expect. Next, I put together a budget for them that detailed all their income, their expenses, and how this service fit nicely within their monthly finances.

Once I had all my material together, I asked to sit down with them and discuss my concerns and what I'd like to see happen. At first, I got the typical response, but once I laid out the financial proof that they could afford it, they couldn't argue with me any longer. They now have the help they need and the added benefit is that they really enjoy the two girls who come each week. Not only do they perform their tasks, but they also sit down for a cup of coffee with Mom and Dad each time and provide a little social stimulation. Now my folks look forward to the girls' visits more than anything. —*Carla*

HAVING THE DISCUSSION

At this point, you should be ready to approach your loved one and get the ball rolling. It is normal to be nervous, scared, or worried about his or her reaction and how it might affect your relationship. Having the discussion with your senior about the fact that he or she is aging and unable to properly care for himself or herself any longer can be uncomfortable and emotional. It can be especially difficult for children who have to face parents who have always been the authority figures in their life for the dreaded "talk." Fortunately, if you've done the previously suggested work and follow the suggestions here, you may be surprised at how well your elder listens to you and find that any resistance begins to melt away.

The Best Location for the Discussion

Surprisingly, many people give little thought as to the setting in which the discussion happens. That is understandable if, in the middle of a situation or crisis, you feel it's necessary to begin mentioning that things need to change now. The location and atmosphere you choose to have such a private, intimate, and potentially life-changing conversation can make all the difference to the outcome. For instance, if you and your brother have been talking about moving Dad to an assisted living facility, don't bring it up to him while dining in a nice restaurant for his birthday. It's likely the discussion will not go well.

When selecting the location, make sure your senior is relaxed, comfortable, and feels safe. It's also a good idea to decide on a setting where your loved one can retreat if necessary, gather his or her emotions, and calm down. However, it's important not only that your elder is at ease but that all other parties are as well. If your mother is a hoarder and being in her home makes you tense and upset, then the conversation will probably reflect those feelings.

Think about where you can best achieve your goal of comfort and privacy. Here are some thoughts when choosing that location.

- Is there plenty of room, and are there comfortable chairs for all participants to sit?

- Will there be outside interferences, such as children rushing in or dogs jumping on people?

- Can everyone be heard without raising voices?

- Is it private enough that participants can express their emotions without embarrassment?

- Are there any time constraints on occupying the space?

The Best Time for the Discussion

The ideal time frame for having any discussions is before your loved one begins to show signs of needing help. But frankly, the subject rarely comes up until there have been symptoms or incidents indicating that help is already needed. Considering the timing of the discussion is equally as important as the location. Ensure that all participants are relaxed, able to say what's on their minds, and don't feel rushed or pressured. The following dos and don'ts will help you determine the best time to engage your senior.

Dos

- Pick a date and time when all members can easily be available for the discussion.

- Make sure you have all contributors updated on details and that they understand the goals of the meeting before setting the date.

- If your senior brings the subject up first, let the conversation unfold at that time and then suggest a family meeting as well.

Don'ts

- Meet during a crisis unless absolutely necessary. Delay the discussion until everyone has a chance to digest what has happened and all the details are clear.

- Engage your loved one if they aren't feeling well.

- Suggest meeting before you have time to fully prepare and practice what you're going to say.

How to Approach the Subject

Your method of approaching the subject can determine whether or not your senior feels ambushed or is shocked that you even feel the conversation is necessary. It is ideal if you can bring the subject up slowly rather than diving right in. Try switching places with your loved one and imagine how he or she might like to be approached. Have you seen signs that your elder is already aware that assistance is needed, or does he or she seem to feel fully capable and might be offended that you would suggest otherwise? Your approach needs to offer insight to and welcome contribution from your loved one. The fact is, your loved one may already know something is happening, so think about comments that might break the ice before blurting anything out.

- "Mom, we would like to spend a few moments to get your input on a couple of things we've noticed recently."

- "I've been struggling to get over here to help you lately. I've researched some ideas on services that help people around the house and would like your opinion on them."

- "Dad, you've mentioned a few times that you have been having difficulties with some activities. Can you explain this further for us? We'd like to see what we could do to help."

If you can get your loved one talking about what has been a problem or concern, it will make it easier for you to admit that you've seen the same thing and have been thinking about ways to resolve the matter. By now, your elder will have shown an openness to a discussion or not. Depending on the outcome, you may even be able to adjust your presentation of the facts accordingly. Not knowing how your senior will react can be nerve wracking. Here are some steps you can take to know your material before delivering it to your loved one.

- Prepare a script if it would make you more comfortable.

- Practice your words. Stand in front of a mirror, and say it over and over again until you feel at ease and won't worry about losing your focus.

- Make notes to have on hand if you're concerned about forgetting anything.

- Keep your comments precise, and don't wander off topic.

- Organize documents in the order in which you want to discuss them.

- Ask your loved one for his or her thoughts.

- Remember that your elder has a right to express himself or herself and that your loved one may have valid points to consider.

- Listen to everyone's comments before responding.

- Don't allow the meeting to devolve into a complaint session.

- Don't engage in power plays.

- Understand that there may not be a conclusion with just one meeting, but that it may take several before anything is decided.

I was so worried about how to approach my dad when I wanted him to move out of his home to an assisted living community closer to me. He was an hour away, and with my own family, kids to drive around all day, and a part-time job, it was hard to find the time to not only check up on him but to also have any quality time together. Our visits mainly consisted of me going over for a couple of hours on the weekend and grocery shopping for him or running any other errands he might need.

One night, while lying in bed and stressing over how I could handle this, I had a brilliant idea. I'm his only child, and he loves me dearly. He's always said there wasn't anything he wouldn't do for me. So I decided to use this to my advantage. I called him the next day and set up a time for us to go out for coffee. I took him to his favorite coffee shop, where we could sit in the corner on a big comfy couch and enjoy our treats.

I began the conversation by talking about my life and how the kids keep me so busy. I also shared the fact that my husband's hours were cut back and that I was working more to make up for the difference. As I imagined, he listened and grew concerned for us. His first reaction was to offer us money, but I said no. I told him that the best thing he could was to move to a community near our home. With him living closer to us, I wouldn't have to spend my weekends driving over and doing chores, I could visit more frequently to help and we'd have more free time for things like having coffee or going to lunch. I also pointed out that his grandkids would be able to ride their bikes over to see him and that he could come over for dinner at least once a week. I took his hand and told him I wouldn't ask him to do anything he didn't want to do, but that I really needed and wanted to be closer to him. His protective nature took over, and he agreed to spend the next weekend at our house so that we could visit the community together.

I'm happy to say that this worked out wonderfully. Dad moved a couple of months after our discussion, and he's happy he did it. We spend much more quality time together, and he feels proud of himself that he was able to do something to help me. *—Faith*

How to Respond to Pushback from Your Loved One

No matter how well prepared you are, there will be comments or questions that you wished you had a response for. Think about how often you looked back at a conversation and wished you'd thought of saying this or that, but you were simply caught off guard. Here are a few examples of common statements you might hear when a loved one is resistant to any change and how you might answer them.

- *"There's nothing wrong with me, and I don't need help."*

  "Nobody is saying anything is wrong with you. It's a normal part of life to eventually need some help. All we want to do it make sure your life is as easy and enjoyable as possible. Please let us tell you what we've noticed and how we think we might be able to ease our minds and make sure you're healthy, happy, and safe for a long time to come."

- *"I can't afford help."*

  "I don't think that's true. I've done some research and here is the pricing. I believe that, if we carefully plan for your care or apply for any financial resources available, you can comfortably afford . . . (whatever resource you are hoping to put in to place)."

- *"Why can't you take care of me?"*

  "Mom, there's nothing I would like more than that, but the facts are (insert your information), and it just isn't possible. But what I can do is make sure that we find the best care possible for you. I will always be available for you to talk to me about anything you need or any concerns you have, I just won't be doing the actual caregiving."

- *"You don't care about me at all." "I'm not going to do it." "Why don't you love me?"*

"That's not true. I'm doing this because I do love you, and I want what's best for you and for all of us. I want to know how you feel about these solutions, and I want you to help me make the best choices, but something needs to change whether you are willing to help or not. These are your options, and one of them will be the action taken. I would like for you to have a say in the matter and what decisions we make."

CAREGIVER SURVIVAL TIP

Our elders grew up recognizing certain professionals as authority figures—such as doctors, religious leaders, police officers, and firemen—and they respected and listened to them without question. If these experts told them they needed to do something, it was likely your loved ones would not hesitate to do as instructed.

However, it doesn't always work that way when we, their family, tell them we have concerns and want to make changes in their life. Often, they react as though we can't possibly know what we're talking about. We're just their kids, and they know better.

A successful tactic to take when speaking with your senior about major changes is to ask one of these experts to be the bad guy. Request to meet ahead of time, in person and without your loved one, to discuss your worries and ask if the expert will support you by initiating the need for change. Usually it is your senior's doctor who has the greatest experience and intimate knowledge related to your loved one and who can persuade your elder most easily to allow assistance into the home or make a move to a new home.

Using someone else as the messenger of bad news allows you to be the knight in shining armor. Once the shock wears off and your loved one begins to feel angry or upset over the situation, you can step in and say, "I know this is hard on you and that you don't want to do it. But it has to happen, and I promise that I'm going to find the best caregiver or the best community possible. Don't worry. I love you and will do everything possible to make this a good experience."

This approach can often save family members from bearing all the responsibility of insisting on changes and the negative feelings your loved one may express over them.

CHAPTER 8

Making the Right Decision

Facing the challenge of handling your loved one's future can bring up emotions like guilt, fear, or anger—even in the strongest of personalities. The individual who has taken the initiative in addressing care issues and encouraging the decision to make changes is usually the one closest emotionally to her senior. She has been the person who has been checking in regularly, on-call for emergencies, or providing care herself, and it can feel as if she is giving up and letting her elder down when it's suggested that it's time for another form of assistance.

Asking loved ones to welcome change or move to a new environment can be uncomfortable or even distressing. It's likely they have developed schedules, routines, and habits that aren't easily altered; and when they are most vulnerable, you are insisting they must listen to you and perhaps go against their own wishes. Suddenly they are expected to allow strangers in to their home, honor someone else's timetable, and follow instructions that may be confusing or that they don't agree with. Or they must adjust to a new home setting where they will have to make different friends, trust unknown caregivers, and learn the community rules.

It's been said by eldercare professionals that when you disrupt a senior's life—especially if you relocate her—and even if she is receptive to the idea of change, she will decline physically and mentally, even if it's just a small degree. You have to hold your breath and hope she will rebound quickly and start to flourish under the new conditions. Don't worry; a decline is almost always a temporary condition. But the last thing you want is to realize that you've made a mistake and have to start all over again.

APPROACHING YOUR DECISION

In any situation, there are factors you can control and others you cannot. It's understandable that, when making important care decisions, you want to cover every possible need and do your best to prevent anything bad from happening. The following suggestions can help you decide whether you are heading down the right path or need to reconsider your choices.

- **Don't be afraid to ask yourself the hard questions.** Decide whether you are making accurate judgments about your loved one's condition and what he or she requires. Sometimes you need an unbiased set of eyes to help you see clearly. Don't be afraid to ask for others' opinions.

- **Take into consideration your own needs and those of other family members besides your loved one.** Focusing only on your senior, other relationships can suffer. It can also lead to the deterioration of your mental or physical health to the point where you need care yourself and you focus less on your loved one. There's a reason caregivers often pass away before their loved ones do. Consider that, when healthy and independent, your senior would never want to put you through this.

When my family was looking for an assisted living community for our mom, we had the vision of her living in a large center, making new friends, and enjoying all the activities. Unfortunately, we found that after she settled in, Mom never came out of her apartment. She said she was afraid she would get lost in the community, and she was too shy or nervous to ask for help. Over the first month, she became so lonely and depressed that we knew something drastic had to change or she would continue to suffer.

When I spoke with her doctor, he asked if we had looked into any smaller care homes. I didn't know anything about them, so he handed me a couple of brochures for homes he provides house visits for and suggested I take a look. The first was nice, but I didn't care for the owner. But the minute I walked into the second one, I knew it was the place for Mom.

We moved her a week later and there was an immediate connection between Mom, the owner, and her staff. However, Mom was still quiet and wanted to stay in her room. She asked if a caregiver would bring her meals to her so she wouldn't have to go to the dining room table. They did, but what was remarkable is that the caregivers would take turns going in and sitting with Mom and talking about her life while she ate. After a week or so, Mom started venturing out of her room and looking for the girls so she could talk to someone. Once that happened, she also encountered the other residents, realized it was like living with her family, and she began to relax.

I'm happy and relieved to say the Mom has recovered her spirit, is eating what everyone else eats, and is doing well. I wish I had talked to more people about some of the choices I was making before rushing ahead. I thought I knew what was best, and in this case I made a huge mistake. Thankfully, I realized it early on and corrected it. *—Polly*

- The earlier you put support services in place, the more likely you can extend your loved one's independence and overall well-being. Waiting until a problem occurs or until your senior is unable to welcome changes can make things more difficult. View care as a means of protecting your loved one's lifestyle rather than damaging it.

- **Listen to your heart.** Caregivers often say they knew immediately when they were making the right choice. If a resource or community feels wrong or uncertain to you, pay attention, and continue investigating additional possibilities until you find one you feel comfortable with.

- **Accept that your relationship with your senior may be altered, at least for a while.** It's not uncommon for loved ones to project their fear, anxiety, or anger onto the person trying to help them. Often this is only temporary, but you have to stay strong.

- **Consider some decisions to be temporary solutions.** While it's reasonable to want to make one decision and have it be the solution for the remainder of your elder's life, that may not be feasible. It's more likely that from time to time you will have to reassess and make adjustments as your loved one continues to decline and his or her needs change. This doesn't mean that you have made any mistakes, but only that some things are beyond your control.

KNOWING WHEN TO COMPROMISE

Knowing when to compromise, finding the common middle ground between opposing points of view, and hoping that both parties will find the solution acceptable can be the key to resolving an issue and preserving relationships. In eldercare, there can be instances when you may have to make a concession with your loved one in order to move

Never in my wildest dreams did I think my Dad would refuse to talk to me. We had been so close all my life. He came to every baseball game I've ever played, was the best man at my wedding, and I named my first-born son after him. For 56 years he's not only been my father; he's also been my best friend.

As Dad has grown older, he's struggled with his memory. Things have gotten much worse, and he was finally diagnosed with Alzheimer's disease. He's still able to recognize family and seems to know his way around the house, but recently he's been getting confused and lost outside. Several times, when he's gone to get the mail, he's gotten turned around and ended up knocking on neighbors' doors. With a heavy heart, I realized that he needed to move to a community where he couldn't wander off and possibly hurt himself.

He was furious that I even suggested he leave his home. For the first time in my life, Dad yelled at me and called me names. I was devastated. I tried for a week to convince him why this was a good idea, but he wouldn't even look at me. When I picked him up and drove him to the memory care center, he refused to say good-bye and turned his back to me. Over the next two days, he wouldn't see me or cooperate with the staff. It was horrible. They eventually asked me to stay away for a week so that they could try to bond with him and get him through his anger. That seemed to do the trick. The next time I came, he seemed to have forgotten that he had been angry.

I know I was doing what was best for Dad, but that was one of the most difficult things I've ever done. *—Curtis* forward. Otherwise, the entire objective of seeking care can come to an abrupt halt. It is better to concede on smaller, less important matters in order to succeed on critical issues.

It can be a double-edged sword when your loved ones are still highly functioning and involved in the decision-making process regarding their care. While you may be pleased they are relatively independent and can voice their desires, it can be frustrating when those desires don't match what you feel needs to happen. Out of respect, you may even ask yourself what right you have to impose your will on them. The following questions can help you identify how much and when you should compromise.

- **Have you had a discussion with your loved one about his or her vision of the future?** If you have made decisions without involving your loved one, and the decisions are not in accordance with his or her wishes, you may need to alter them and compromise to reach a common ground.

- **Is your senior willing to compromise on that vision to give you more peace of mind that he or she is being taken care of?** You may be surprised to learn that if your senior feels listened to and not in danger of losing control over his or her life, your loved one may be more willing to accept your recommendations. If you ask him or her to compromise, however, you must be willing to do the same.

- **Are your suggestions reasonable?** Have you done your research and feel confident your proposals are realistic? If, for instance, you are insisting that your parents hire a live-in caregiver, is there a private room where the caregiver can sleep and keep his or her personal property? When flaws in your thinking are pointed out, you might need to rethink your plan.

- **If your loved one is resistant, do the objections make sense?** Consider your senior's opinions and decide whether you may be overreacting to them. Are you making fear-based decisions? Could there be other solutions? If your senior is being reasonable in his or her protests, try to reach a compromise.

- **Can you take baby steps toward higher levels of care, or do you need to make immediate and significant changes right now?** This consideration depends on your loved one's condition and what he or she is capable of handling. If your mother simply needs help with household chores and you are suggesting she move to an assisted living community, chances are she will be resistant. Agreeing to a cleaning service instead may be a good compromise. But if your father has had a massive stroke and can no longer function without significant assistance, you are being reasonable in suggesting he move to an assisted living facility, a compromise may not be possible or desirable.

- **Has your loved one continually reneged on solutions he or she approved after you reached agreement?** If there is a pattern of agreeing to certain actions and then refusing or attempting to renegotiate, recognize that your senior is stalling or sabotaging your efforts, and let him or her know that you will no longer compromise.

- **Is the situation yes or no?** If you can honestly say there are no other choices available, such as your father requiring constant supervision and support but you and your family cannot afford 24-hour care, there is no room for compromise. In this case, the answer is no, you can't afford private care, and yes, you need to move him to a less expensive assisted living group home.

- **Is your loved one a danger to himself or herself or to others?** You cannot compromise when there is a concern that someone might be in danger.

I was raised in a very strict household where my parents always had the last say. Dad ruled with a heavy hand and even when he passed away, I still respected Mom and followed her instructions or honored her wishes regarding everything.

When the house started to become too much for her to handle on her own, my kids and I would pitch in and help her, but as they got older, it became harder to dedicate that kind of time. I would try and get Mom to let me hire someone to help and she would always agree, but when they showed up to do the work, she'd complain about them and fire them.

Later on, when Mom fell and broke her hip, she needed rehabilitation. The doctor told her he would write a prescription so that she could continue physical therapy on her own once she left the rehabilitation center. She told everyone how she would work hard on getting her strength back, but after a few sessions she refused to schedule any more.

Every time I tried to discuss it, she would firmly put me in my place and tell me that she was still the parent and I won't be telling her what to do. Because she refused to accept help or do the work necessary to stay healthy, she began to get very fragile. I finally decided I needed to get my courage up and make some decisions, whether she approved or not. She needed to move to a place where they could watch over her and take care of anything she needed. I made plans for us to look at some communities several times, but she always cancelled at the last minute with some flimsy excuse. After three times, I told her that I was going to go on my own and pick the place for her. By then, I had no patience left.

Mom never participated in looking at apartments or talking with the staff. She thought if she ignored it, the move would go away. I ended up having to pick the apartment and arrange for the move. Mom went willingly once it was all arranged, but I think she thought she could put me off and I would give up. *–Billie*

DECIDING WHO MAKES THE FINAL DECISION

There can be tremendous pressure and responsibility in making the final decision on eldercare. Ideally, our loved ones would be in a position to make these choices for themselves, but often they are too unsure, in denial, or mentally unable to do so. In these cases, someone else needs to step in and take charge. To determine who will be the most appropriate selection to make these ultimate conclusions, start with the following considerations.

- **Has my loved one expressed his wishes in the past and are they still feasible?** If he is capable of making sound decisions and his desires are reasonable and can be carried out, your senior should have the last word on what eldercare choices are made.

- **Is my loved one too ill to make the decision for himself?** If his health has prevented him from participating in his care, whoever has the legal right to act on his behalf must do so.

- **Is my loved one capable of making rational and sound judgments?** If he suffers from a mental illness or dementia and cannot decide what is in his best interest, his opinion can be requested, but ultimately you, as the representative, must step in and make the decision.

- **How do we decide what to do if the family is not in agreement?** If there is a legal representative, such as a power of attorney or guardian, and he wishes to force that power over the decision-making process, he has the right to do so.

However, if family members want to reach an amiable conclusion, enlist the services of a family mediator to assist you in coming to the best resolution possible.

- **What do we do if no one has legal authority, and our loved one is incapable of making decisions?** You will most likely have to seek guardianship or conservatorship to make decisions on his behalf. A judge will appoint someone on the senior's behalf to make choices for him.

In making eldercare decisions, your first choice should be to include your loved one in the process. If that is not a viable option, then ask whoever has the legal authority to make decisions on your senior's behalf to work through the preceding questions. Sometimes the answer is made clear for you through that process alone.

■■■■■■■■■■   CAREGIVER SURVIVAL TIP   ■■■■■■■■■■

When making decisions for your loved one is so overwhelming that you don't know where to begin, it can be helpful to identify specific steps and create a system to guide you through the process. Here is a model for systematically making informed decisions.

Identify the issue. Define the problem using specific details, such as "Dad has left the stove on three times in the last month." By isolating individual issues, it will allow you to focus more clearly.

Gather information. By getting all the data you can, you will be making decisions based on facts and not on assumptions, emotions, or opinions.

Ascertain and assess your options. Brainstorm and identify as many options as possible. Then consider the short-term and long-term consequences of each and compare them.

Develop a strategy. Speak with anyone involved in the care of your loved one and create a step-by-step blueprint for initiating and carrying out the plan.

Take action. Determine which option is best, and do what is necessary to put it in place.

Evaluate the results. Give the plan a reasonable period of time and then assess the outcome. Keep an open mind about altering the strategy, if necessary. Try another option if your plan is not working as anticipated.

CHAPTER 9

Special Considerations for Care

The responsibilities of providing care can seem complicated and never ending. They can be particularly challenging if your loved one has special requirements, such as home dialysis equipment or a room monitor to enable listening and increased security in another room or area of the house. These extraordinary circumstances can involve caring for a loved one of any age and demand that you accept outcomes you had hoped to avoid or do things you had never expected to have to do. Such situations can break even the most dedicated and determined of caregivers.

Because there is a great deal of emotion and commitment involved in your relationship with your loved one, the thought of not following through or performing above and beyond what is reasonably required may seem unacceptable. At first, you may not even realize how much you've taken on. But at some point, there's a good chance that you will need to receive specialized training, bring in professional assistance, or accept that you are not capable of managing the situation and must relinquish your role as primary caregiver. This can leave you feeling inadequate or that you have failed, but you cannot be expected to intuitively know how to handle your loved one's care.

The first step is in acknowledging that you are managing care for someone who falls into an unusual or high-needs category. By doing so, you will be giving yourself permission to admit that you may not be the right caregiver, don't want to be the caregiver, or need additional help in providing elevated levels of care.

This chapter will help you to understand the debilitating conditions your loved one may be facing and to determine your capability to be able to care for him or her.

THE SPECIAL CARE NEEDS OF A YOUNGER PERSON

In situations where your young loved one will need long-term care—such as being born with a condition like cerebral palsy or having been in an accident and suffering from a traumatic brain injury—most parents believe that their child will receive the best and most attentive support at home. If you are in such a situation, you may have the impression that you must provide all the care yourself and that, if you don't, you are abandoning your child. However, there are instances where it can be best to turn a child's care over to others. For instance, perhaps your child has reached a point in life where it would be beneficial to move to an environment that will encourage him or her to grow as an individual.

If your loved one is a senior, the need for assistance usually stems from the normal cognitive or physical decline of aging, and the focus is on providing care during the final days, months, or years. But if your loved one is young and suffers from severe physical or mental incapacities, it's probable that care will be required for decades.

While you still have the same options for providing care that exist with an older person, consider the following questions.

- *Are you fully capable of providing for your young loved one's health care needs?*

   ☐ Are you able to perform objectively as a caregiver?

☐ Do you need specialized training to meet her needs?

☐ Are you able to dedicate yourself to her care, or will you be torn between working and caregiving for many years to come?

☐ Will you grow too old to provide care?

☐ Do you have your own health concerns?

• *Will your loved one receive appropriate social stimulation for her age?*

☐ If she is confined to the home, will she be able to interact with others of the same age group?

☐ What steps can you take to ensure she reaches development milestones for good emotional and mental health? For instance, you may need to enroll her in young adult day care or a school for those with special care needs.

• *If this is a permanent condition, could she benefit from moving to a young adult assisted living community?*

☐ Is there a possibility that she could finish school or learn a vocation while living in a supervised environment?

☐ Would your young loved one gain from being around others her age that are also living with challenges?

☐ Will moving to a community allow her to grow as an individual?

• *Have you taken necessary steps to provide for her care if or when something happens to you?*

☐ Do you have the necessary legal documents, like an estate plan, indicating your wishes and how you'd like your loved one to be cared for if you were incapacitated or deceased?

☐ Have you introduced your young one to the outside world so that it wouldn't be traumatic if you were no longer her caregiver? For instance, does she go to a young adult care community while you take a respite? Or does she regularly visit and stay with other family members who might take over caregiving duties?

What must also be considered is how to go about finding resources that specialize in young adults with care needs. Here are some suggestions that may offer a great deal of help to you as you make decisions for your young loved one.

- **Ask professionals such as doctors, social workers, or support groups if they know of organizations or communities that specialize in younger clients or residents.** By reaching out, broadening your contacts with those who manage the care of younger people, and developing a sphere of expert resources, your options of finding the appropriate support will be better.

- **If you need to move your young loved one to a care community, do not rule out traditional assisted living facilities.** Although you may not be able to find a specialized community that focuses on young adults, traditional facilities may still be an option. Explore whether they are willing to accept a resident under the ages 55–65. Ask the community director about the resident population and whether there are any younger residents. Inquire as to what programs the community can offer younger residents and what type of stimulation and socialization opportunities they would receive.

TRAUMATIC BRAIN INJURY

Traumatic brain injury (TBI) occurs when an external force—usually the result of a violent blow or a jolt to the head or body from a car

My daughter, Shelby, is 32 years old and suffers from debilitating seizures. Although she appears young and healthy, is capable of driving, and works to support herself, she can suffer a grand mal seizure at any moment. When that happens, she is often crippled for weeks, if not months, afterwards. Shelby has an assistance dog specially trained to warn her 20 minutes ahead of time when she is going to seize, and hopefully she can get off the road or to a safe setting and let others know what will be happening.

Shelby has always lived with my husband and me, but we are getting older and it's hard on us when she has a seizure. It's difficult to care for her over a long period of time. We have discussed this matter with Shelby, as well as the fact that she should be living on her own and interacting with younger people more. We decided that it would be best if she moved to a place where she could receive care during those times she needed to recover from her attacks. After much research and touring communities, Shelby finally found a large assisted living center that allowed people under the age of 55 with disabilities. The number of seniors still outweighs the number of younger people there, but there will be at least a dozen or more individuals living there and many of the staff members are closer to her age. It's hard to ask Shelby to move out. I wish we could have her with us forever, but it's worth it to know that when she's incapable of caring for herself, the staff is there for her. –*Delores*

accident, sports injury, or act of violence—causes brain dysfunction. TBI can cause mild to severe symptoms that may last a relatively brief period of time or can be permanent and cause serious disability. These injuries can lead to a variety of prolonged or permanently altered levels of consciousness.

- **Vegetative state.** This usually results from widespread damage to the brain. The individual is unaware of his or her surroundings, but may open his or her eyes, make sounds, move about, or respond to stimuli.

- **Minimally conscious state.** There may be some evidence of self-awareness or an awareness of the individual's environment.

- **Locked-in syndrome.** There is an awareness of his or her surroundings, but the individual is awake yet unable to speak or move.

- **Coma.** The individual is unconscious, unaware of anything, and unable to respond to any stimuli.

- **Brain death.** If taken off of life support, the individual will die.

The level and type of care your loved one may require after suffering a traumatic brain injury will depend on the level of consciousness as well as his or her physical/mental needs. Some of the more serious symptoms include the following:

- seizures, often called posttraumatic epilepsy

- fluid buildup, infections, blood vessel damage, and nerve damage to the brain

- intellectual problems such as lack of judgment, poor reasoning capabilities, or difficulty concentrating

- communication challenges like difficulty with speech or writing, inability to organize thoughts or ideas, and problems expressing emotion

- behavioral and emotional changes including difficulty with self-control, trouble in social situations, and lack of empathy for others

- sensory issues such as impaired eye–hand coordination, blind spots, double vision, and trouble with balance or dizziness

- increased risk of brain diseases such as Alzheimer's and Parkinson's resulting from the degeneration of brain cells

Our daughter was a passenger in a car that was hit broadside in an intersection. She was 37 years old at the time and suffered severe traumatic brain injury. For the past nine years, she has been in a vegetative state, but I believe she knows who I am and when I'm with her. My husband and her doctors disagree with me.

I found myself unable to send her to a care community after the accident. I couldn't bear the thought of her living alone without her mother, and we can afford the private care at home. Since the accident, I have cared for her during the day, and we have a home health aide who works at night so I can sleep.

This has caused a great deal of stress and contention in my marriage. My husband recently told me that he would move out and move on with his life without me if I did not agree to transfer our daughter to a skilled nursing facility. He feels that she will not know the difference, and we will be able to live our lives knowing she is taken care of. He's close to retirement and wants a more normal life.

We don't know how long she might live under these circumstances. It could be another year, or another 20 years. I had to make the most difficult choice of my life and agreed to move her to a facility. She has been there for six months now and nothing has changed. I realize that having me with her every day will not bring her back to me, and my husband no longer feels like he's lost both his daughter and his wife. By having her in a community, we are able to work on rebuilding our life together. —*Stephanie*

As a caregiver for a loved one with TBI, you may be faced with providing long-term care for someone who suffers serious physical, mental, and emotional problems. Seek counsel from experts to determine if you are the right person to provide care for that individual or what other options you should consider to manage your loved one's needs.

ALZHEIMER'S DISEASE AND OTHER RELATED DEMENTIAS

When memory issues develop into dementia, your loved one will need more specialized care as the condition worsens over time. Eventually, your senior's needs may exceed what you can provide at home or what an assisted living community is willing to manage in its facility.

Scenarios that may indicate that your loved one needs specialized care and cannot remain in his or her current living situation include the following:

- disorientation
- an inability to understand or remember who or where he or she is
- failure to recognize family
- tendency to wander, and therefore at risk of becoming lost
- inability to recognize danger
- the indication of behavioral or emotional problems
- an inability to perform the majority of ADL without assistance
- a risk for trips, falls, or accidents
- being in a care situation that no longer meets your loved one's needs
- the need for full-time supervision

If you find yourself unable to handle the care for a loved one in the later stages of dementia, there are expert memory care communities dedicated to those with these problems. Some existing communities have also recognized the growing need and are committing areas for this specific type of resident. These facilities have staff trained in dementia care and can meet specific challenges such as redirecting behaviors, providing reassurance, and calming agitated residents.

PARKINSON'S DISEASE AND SIMILAR CONDITIONS

When dealing with a long-term progressive illness such as Parkinson's disease, muscular dystrophy (MLS), or Lou Gehrig's disease (ALS), families must consider how it will progress over time and what modifications will need to be made to the person's care as a result. This is where researching options and planning ahead can make a difference to how well you and your loved one handle care options and adjust to the changes as they occur.

Often, these conditions remain stable for years, and the progression allows enough time to tackle each new requirement as it appears. People with Parkinson's disease can live as long as those without it, but over time they will have an ever-increasing need for assistance. On the other hand, people with a condition such as ALS are expected to live only three to five years after diagnosis. The condition progresses more rapidly than others and may require more frequent changes to the care plan.

It is important to learn as much as possible about your loved one's condition and then address the management of the symptoms over his expected life span. The following steps can help you identify how you might prepare for his present and future care needs.

- **Seek a professional diagnosis.** Understand what you and your loved one are dealing with. Don't assume that it's

stress, that he is overly tired, or that he has some other condition that would cause similar symptoms when it could
possibly be a stroke, a head injury, or Parkinson's disease.
If his physical or mental ailments are long lasting and not
improving, it is likely that there is something more serious
going on.

- **Learn about the progression of the condition.** Ask yourself
  whether you are facing increasing care needs for your loved

When my wife was diagnosed with Parkinson's disease, we sat
down and had a long discussion about what that meant to our
marriage and our lives. I am not and have never been a very
nurturing person. Although I wanted to honor my marriage
vows, I think we both realized there would come a time when
things might need to change drastically.

For many years, we handled her condition without much
assistance. When it got to the point that she shouldn't be
alone, we hired a professional agency for those occasions
when I would be away. Then, one day, something terrible
happened. I had a stroke. Although I recovered almost completely, it shook me up. By now, my wife was having some early
signs of dementia related to her Parkinson's, and I thought
to myself, "What happens if I have another stroke?" I wasn't
worried about what would happen to her, I was afraid that
she wouldn't realize I needed help and call 911. She would
probably just go about her day, and I would lie on the floor
and die.

I made the decision that we would move together into a
luxury assisted living community. I will keep the house, and
when she passes on or doesn't care if I'm with her any longer,
I will move back home. I love my wife, but I love myself just
as much. *–Keith*

one over the next two years or the next twenty years. Consider issues such as whether you will simply need to provide basic assistance with activities of daily living or if it is likely to become more serious over time and you will be required to hire health care professionals to provide skilled medical care as your loved one's body ceases to function properly. Develop a working timeline of what you can expect for planning purposes.

- **Create a plan that determines what and when resources should be put in place to ensure that the needs of everyone involved are being met.** Conduct research on resources, care options, and financial planning. Keep in mind that the plan needs to be flexible enough to change for any unexpected events.

- **Have an open and honest discussion with your loved one as to what the future looks like and what he can realistically expect.** Use the information you've gained by familiarizing yourself with his condition, and describe what types of care you anticipate needing to put in place as his needs progress. Explain whether you feel capable of meeting those demands yourself or if you will want to seek assistance from others.

FEEDING TUBES, TRACHEOTOMY TUBES, AND OTHER MEDICAL DEVICES

As your loved one's body begins to shut down, there will be a need for a variety of medical devices to assist with functions your senior is no longer able to perform. Family members can receive training and, if willing, perform duties to monitor, clean, replace parts, or handle other equipment necessities.

Gear that family caregivers might need to manage include the following items.

- **Durable medical equipment.** This equipment might include hospital beds, lifts, wheelchairs, scooters, and toilet or bath chairs.

- **Oxygen tanks.** Tanks, tubing, and cannula (the device that is placed into the nostrils to deliver a mixture of air and oxygen) are easily cared for and common in aiding the elderly or those with problems breathing.

- **Ostomy pouches.** These pouches, used to collect body waste, require regular changing, after which the surgically created opening in the body must be cleansed.

- **Catheters.** This is a flexible tube inserted through a narrow opening into a body cavity for the removal of fluids.

- **Feeding tubes.** There are several different types of feeding tubes, and, depending on which type required, you may be able to care for it yourself or it may require a skilled professional.

Equipment that family caregivers may consider too difficult to handle or that require skilled professionals to operate include the following items.

- **Mechanical ventilator.** This is a tube inserted into the windpipe to assist an individual with breathing.

- **Tracheotomy tube.** This is a ventilator (breathing) tube placed through a surgically made hole in the front of the person's neck and down into the windpipe to help with breathing.

- **Suctioning equipment.** This is a device used to remove liquids, such as mucus or serum, and gases from the body cavity and airways.

Not every caregiver wants to perform these tasks or handle this sort of medical equipment. When considering who will provide care for your loved one, you will need to discuss specifics with the potential caregiver and ensure that the person is trained and willing to manage these types of equipment. If considering an assisted living community, be aware that not all communities will allow or manage certain pieces of medical equipment.

DIALYSIS

If your loved one has kidney disease and requires dialysis, he or she will either need assistance with home dialysis equipment or be able to visit a dialysis clinic for treatment. Both can be time consuming and difficult.

Home dialysis allows your loved one to receive treatment in the comfort of his or her own home and offers more flexibility of scheduling. Anyone involved in the treatment must commit to effective time management. The following considerations can help you determine if home dialysis will be an option you and your loved one wish to pursue.

- Home dialysis allows the patient to decide when and where it's most convenient. For example, he or she could dialyze in the living room while watching television with family members or at night while sleeping.
- The equipment must be clean and easily accessible.
- Home dialysis may require specific plumbing and/or electrical modifications to the home.

- There may be additional costs to the household budget, such as higher water and utility bills.

- Both the caregiver and patient must receive intensive training, which can take from two to five weeks to complete.

- The caregiver must have adequate manual dexterity and vision to perform dialysis-related tasks and operate the equipment.

- You must also realize that, as the caregiver, your schedule will need to be adjusted to match your loved one's home dialysis requirements.

If you feel uncomfortable committing to the option of home dialysis or have trouble finding a home health agency willing to assist, there is the option of receiving treatment at a dialysis center. This includes the following benefits.

- Your loved one will be surrounded by health care professionals trained to watch over patients who are receiving treatment.

- You will be able to leave your loved one at the clinic and go back to work, run errands, or take some time for yourself.

- It eliminates the need for training, equipment, and supplies in the home and the stress of providing dialysis care.

Regardless of whether your loved one is receiving dialysis at home or in a clinic, as the caregiver, you will need to ensure that your senior adheres to a prescribed treatment that includes following specific dialysis timing, diet, and medications.

BED-BOUND PATIENTS

Bed-bound patients require around the clock attention that often involves medical practices or treatments. Some of the major duties that you will need to understand and be willing to perform before accepting responsibility for your bed-bound senior include the following:

- Your loved one's position must be changed every two hours to relieve pressure on the back, buttocks, and hips to avoid bedsores.

- You must perform daily or twice daily skin checks to detect skin breakdown that will result in bedsores. It is especially important to wash the genital area because bacteria tend to collect there.

- You need to brush and floss your loved one's teeth or assist him or her with the process.

- You may need to assist with eating and drinking liquids. You may be required to feed or hydrate your loved one if he or she cannot do it alone. If your senior has a feeding tube, you will need to manage any intake of nutrition and hydration through the tube.

- You must monitor and assist with breathing such as changing positions, clearing lungs and airways, or utilizing oxygen therapy equipment.

- You will need to assess his or her pain through visual or verbal clues and manage it with advice and instructions from your loved one's medical or hospice team, including the use of medications or proper positioning.

- You may need to handle the elimination of body waste. This can involve adult diapers, ostomy pouches, or catheters.

BEHAVIORAL ISSUES

With many physical or mental conditions, there can be a drastic change in personality and behaviors. This is especially true with traumatic brain injuries and dementia. This can all be very stressful for the caregiver and family members. Depending on the part of the brain that is damaged and the severity, your loved one may experience personality changes, memory and judgment deficits, lack of impulse control, and poor concentration.

Here are common behavioral issues and actions that may help you to manage them.

- **Rage, anger and yelling.** Try to identify the cause and rectify the matter. For example, if your loved one is showing distress over chronic pain or anger about being incontinent, try not to take it personally.

- **Swearing, offensive language, and inappropriate comments.** Divert your loved one's attention to another subject or talk about the good old days and engage his long-term memory skills. If diversion and reengagement doesn't work, you may have to simply walk away and come back later.

- **Hostile, irritable, or uncooperative attitude.** Attempt to keep your loved one calm, secure, and comfortable by adhering to as normal a routine as possible. Watch for triggers that you can identify and avoid in the future, and do not show frustration or use words or body language that will encourage his behavior. Again, you may have to walk way and approach him again later.

- **Paranoia and hallucinations.** Be as reassuring as possible, because you are not going to be able to convince your loved one he is having a delusion.

My husband had a degenerative brain disease and, as his symptoms began to worsen, he became quite difficult to be around. He'd always been the type of man who needed to be in control, and now I found myself required to jump whenever he asked for anything, no matter how ridiculous or irrational his requests were. I did the best I could to manage the situation, but when he began physically intimidating me, I couldn't handle it any longer. The last straw was when he threw me to the floor and threatened to kill me if I didn't change all of our investments. I locked myself in the bathroom with the phone and called 911.

He was admitted to the behavioral health unit in our local hospital, and it was decided that he would need to move to a memory care community. The damage to his brain was so severe, he would only continue to get worse. There, the medical team would be able to medicate him and manage his behaviors better than I could at home. He was considered dangerous at this point.

I loved my husband, but I had to take steps to protect myself and to give him the level of care he needed.
—Evelyn

- **Physical, emotional, or sexual abuse.** Try talking with your loved one about how his behavior makes you or other caregivers feel. If this does not work, enlist the aid of a counselor, the authorities, or possibly remove your loved one from his place of residence to a setting equipped to handle behavioral problems. Abuse in any form should never be accepted.

- **Obsessive-compulsive behavior.** Contact a mental health professional. Therapy and/or medication may prove helpful.

- **Refusing to shower or manage hygiene.** Do your best to keep your loved one clean. At the same time, consider whether your loved one may be embarrassed or too modest to have a family member clean him. If he has dementia, he may be frightened of the water. While poor eyesight, reduced sense of smell, or memory loss can be among the reasons for this problem, it can also be a method of control. A professional caregiver may need to be hired to manage his hygiene, or you may need to accept that he may no longer meet your definition of cleanliness.

One of the most difficult issues surrounding caregiving is managing those with behavioral issues, whether the person is living independently, with family, or in an assisted living community. It is possible that those providing care will ultimately find themselves unwilling or incapable of handling your loved one's demeanor. Forgive yourself if you or those you originally turned to for support find it is too much and can't follow through on well-intended promises. No matter what the desires are regarding caring for your loved one, remember that everyone has limits. There may come a time when your loved one will require some form of professional assistance or need to be relocated to a behavioral health facility to manage your senior's medications and care.

████████████████   CAREGIVER SURVIVAL TIP   ████████████████

While it is honorable that you may want to provide care for a loved one with special care considerations, there are instances where it might be in everyone's best interests to make other arrangements. If you exhibit or experience any of the following reactions or feelings, find someone you trust to discuss the situation with, like your loved one's medical team or a counselor, and investigate the possibility of turning your senior's care over to another party:

- resentment, anger, or fear toward your loved one
- worry or stress that you cannot perform the tasks required
- extreme dislike or distress toward necessary caregiving duties
- obsessive worries that interrupt sleep and normal day-to-day activities
- loneliness
- helplessness
- suicidal thoughts

CHAPTER 10

Final Words of Advice After Any Change

It would be nice if you could simply assess your loved one's needs, decide what caregiving support should be put in place, carry through with your decisions, and then relax, knowing you've made the right choices. For many families, it doesn't end up being quite that easy. Even when your loved one is receptive to assistance from family members, outside agencies, or moving to an assisted living community, there is often a period of time where he or she will struggle and possibly act out against the changes. Your loved one will need to examine and deal with new and sometimes difficult emotions and feelings, adjust to unfamiliar people providing help, or perhaps discover how to navigate through foreign living arrangements by learning the layout of the community, figuring out the way it operates, and making new friends. No matter how small the change, or how insignificant it may seem to you, your senior may experience a profound reaction to it.

Imagine how difficult this timeframe can be for a family whose loved one is not very receptive or completely against any changes to his or her life or who has dementia and can't understand what is happening. Now get ready for another unanticipated element—you and anyone else involved in your loved one's care may experience similar reactions.

The key to making this period of time successful for all involved is to anticipate and plan for it. The chances are high that you will experience some reaction from your loved one, whether it's physical or emotional. If you are expecting it, you won't be caught off guard and panic when it happens. Just as when you were researching care options, interviewing resources, and bringing the family together to make decisions, you will benefit from understanding what is happening to your loved one. You'll need to educate yourself on ways to deal with your senior's reaction (and yours), and make decisions on how you might handle anything you find concerning.

The "transition period," which is what this stage is commonly referred to, can sometimes be more difficult than the stages you've already managed. If you're not careful, this is when you are at risk of you or your loved one taking all the hard work, commitment, and excellent choices you have made and throwing them out the window.

THE TRANSITION PERIOD

A transition period is the change or passage from one state or stage to another. In the world of caregiving, this might include transitions after each of the following stages:

- monitoring your loved one once you notice he or she needs support

- providing minimal assistance with daily activities

- realizing the need to juggle other commitments in order to provide assistance

- changing working hours to accommodate an increasing need to provide help

- increasing minimal support to higher levels of care, including hands-on assistance such as bathing your loved one or physically escorting him or her as your elder moves about

- hiring outside support when you can no longer meet your senior's needs

- moving your senior in with family or to a care community

Each change, no matter how small or insignificant, can trigger a period of adjustment. Recognizing that you and your loved one are experiencing a reaction to an adjustment can help you slow down, accept that time is needed to adapt, and delay any reactions that might damage or reverse the progress you've made.

COMMON MISTAKES MADE DURING THE TRANSITION

Often, families make errors of judgment that end up prolonging the transition period or perhaps even sabotaging it. Of course, they don't intend to, but it can be difficult for anyone involved in the change to see how their actions might cause more harm than good. Clearly, nobody wants to put changes in place that affect their loved one and then not monitor them to ensure they have the desired results. But how will you know when you are hindering the process? Here are examples of why a transition period might not successfully resolve itself.

- **Participants refuse to accept that the transition will take time.** It always takes some period of time to learn what to expect from the change and adjust accordingly. This includes allowing time for you and your loved one to learn and become comfortable with new routines; allowing caregivers to get to know details about your senior's likes and dislikes in addition to his or her care needs; and

My father was living in an assisted living community. He was an extremely high-fall risk and refused to push his button when he needed assistance. After falling, he would berate the caregivers for not doing a good job. One day the executive director talked with me about my father's needs and the difficulty they were having meeting them. She said he would need to move and suggested a private group home where they could monitor him closely.

Dad was very angry and behaved horribly. In the group home, he was cussing, swinging at the caregivers, and calling everyone names, including me. Within the first week, the owner of the care home said that she was going to have to ask us to move him if he didn't calm down. She said she would give him another week to work through his issues, but that I needed to tell him he would be asked to leave if nothing changed.

In my anger, I told him that he wasn't going back to the assisted living community and he wasn't coming home with me. I'd had enough, and he would be on his own and probably committed to a psych ward if he continued to act this way. I left and refused to take his call that night.

Miraculously, the next morning, when the caregivers went into his room, he was sitting up in bed and greeted them with a friendly hello. He said he would love a cup of coffee, but would they mind giving him a shower first? His entire demeanor had changed overnight. I can't tell you how shocked I was when the owner called me and said that he was behaving like a different man.

I drove over later that morning and Dad greeted me with a sheepish grin. He admitted that he was trying to get them to throw him out and force me to let him live on his own again. He was angry that he needed to be there in the first place, but that if he had to live in a group home this was probably one of the best. He said he felt bad about the horrible way he'd treated the caregivers and apologized to them and the other residents.

I'm pleased to say the Dad lived happily in the home for another 18 months until he passed away. *—Cindy*

developing trust between the caregivers, the loved one, and the family.

- **Family members feel guilty.** Even though they may realize that these changes need to occur and that they are doing the right thing, many family members can act out or behave inappropriately because they feel guilty for turning the care over to another party. For instance, they may be overly critical of the caregivers and look for reasons to make mountains out of molehills.

- **Family members won't leave the care to the caregivers.** The new caregivers must be allowed to do their job. Your loved one needs to bond with them; otherwise, he or she may not grow to depend on and trust in the professionals now handling your senior's care. It is not uncommon for family members to be asked to spend some time away from a caregiving situation so that the appropriate connections can happen.

- **Family members micromanage the care.** In some instances, while family members are willing to let others provide the care, they will monitor every action the caregiver takes or instruct them on how to handle their responsibilities because they feel guilty or untrusting. This can not only instill a sense of resentment but also send the message to your loved one that he or she shouldn't trust the judgment of the caregivers.

- **Family members overreact and decide it's not working too soon.** It's easy for those emotionally involved to jump to the

My elderly mother lives in her own home, but over the past year I visited every day after work to do chores for her or keep her company. I started to feel suffocated because I could never make plans after work, date, or go on a vacation. I spent all my free time with Mom. I decided that I would hire Sharon, a private caregiver, to spend the day with her, and that way I could pop in every couple of days and check in on her.

Looking back, I can see the huge mistake I made from the beginning. My mom was upset that I was bringing someone in to do what she believed was my responsibility. She liked things just the way they were and was trying to make me feel guilty. Well, I did feel guilty, and I continued to visit every night after work to see how things were going. Mom was always complaining that she didn't like the way Sharon did anything, that it wasn't working for her, and that she needed me to redo this or that once I got there.

After talking with Sharon and hearing her feedback, I learned that Mom wouldn't acknowledge or engage with her, refused her help, and waited for me to come over to take care of everything just the way I always have. Sharon and I decided that I would not come by for at least a week, forcing Mom to interact with her. Once I stopped being so available, Mom grew frustrated with me and started letting Sharon help her. It took two more weeks for her to finally accept that Sharon was the only one who would be there on a regular basis and that she needed to accept her assistance. I don't think it would have ever worked out if I hadn't listed to Sharon's side of the story and continued down the same road. *–Monica*

conclusion that a mistake was made. Anxiety and emotions are running high and family members may assume that they have acted too fast, made the wrong decision, or that things were better the way they were before. This happens to those who don't understand there will be a transition and that it's a normal process for everyone concerned.

SUGGESTIONS FOR A SUCCESSFUL TRANSITION

The time it takes for your loved one to transition to a new caregiving situation will be different for everyone. For some, because their senior is willing to accept the changes and eager to adapt, the shift could be a matter of a day or two. For the majority, a normal period of adjustment is expected to take one to two weeks. On the other hand, if your loved one is completely resistant, has dementia, or exhibits behavioral problems, the transition might take weeks or even months. In this case, it might feel like a battle of the wills over who will give in first. The following suggestions will help you prepare for as smooth a transition as possible.

- **Expect the transition to be challenging.** Don't assume everything will go as planned. Allow a learning curve for new caregivers and/or new living arrangements. Accept that your loved one's displeasure over the situation is acceptable if her health and well-being aren't in jeopardy.

- **Acknowledge that the transition period is not just about your loved one.** Everyone involved in your loved one's care or who has an emotional attachment to her may experience difficulty adjusting. Pay attention, encourage open discussions, and acknowledge her feelings, but don't rush to alter anything right away.

- **Set appropriate boundaries with family members, if necessary.** If there are family members who are causing dissention in the care environment and affecting your loved one's transition, you must inform them that they will be asked to stay away until the shift happens.

- **Don't make light of the transition period.** Recognize and honor the emotions and feelings taking place, but try not to succumb to the negative ones. Instead, focus on the positive benefits of the changes made.

- **Understand that your loved one will likely decline slightly physically or mentally in the beginning.** A temporary physical or mental decline is quite common and, in some instances, can require counseling or short-term use of medication to successfully manage mild depression, anxiety, or sadness over the changes made.

- **Give the period of adjustment time.** Change is hard and can make anyone feel overwhelmed or stressed. Generally, these feelings will be temporary. One of the biggest mistakes made is jumping from one change to the next because enough time to settle in was not given.

NO GUILT: YOU DID THE BEST YOU COULD

The one emotion that can derail the best-laid plans is guilt. If you fall into the trap of believing that you haven't done enough, haven't behaved the right way, or haven't done the right thing, you will suffer from feelings of remorse. It's a self-imposed burden that won't result in productive choices.

During your journey with your loved one, you will be forced to make many decisions on his or her behalf as well as for yourself and for others affected by the situation. Many decisions will be perfect; others might be less than desirable, but necessary. There are ways for you avoid beating yourself up. The following suggestions will help you to avoid or overcome this negative and counterproductive emotion.

- **Identify why you're feeling guilty.** Guilt often comes from feeling that you let someone down, that people will be

I come from a very close, traditional Italian family. It was always expected that my mother would live with my family when she couldn't take care of herself any longer. Unfortunately, my husband has health conditions that require a lot of attention, and I can't take care of both of them.

Against her wishes, we moved Mom into an assisted living community. From the start, she complained about everything. She absolutely hated it there. My friend, who's been through this with her mother, told me to give it three months before moving her to another place. I held out for three weeks, but she made me miserable. "This place is horrible. How can you leave me here? I'm so unhappy."

I found several other communities and took her to look at all of them. She hated them all. Finally, I made a decision for her because she refused to pick one. After moving her from the original community to a second one, she had the nerve to tell me that she liked the first community better! I realized that she was not going to like anything because she wanted to move in with me.

I forced myself to wait it out. My friend was right; it took almost three months for her to come around and accept her new home. Now she's fine, but if I'd given in again, she never would have adjusted. –*Brenda*

mad at you, or that they will think less of you. Carefully consider whether your actions were truly wrong. Chances are, you know in your heart that you made the right decisions.

- **Keep in mind that if your feelings of guilt are based on events that might happen in the future, it's worry not guilt.** People often confuse the two. Understand that neither emotion will change the future or prevent something bad from happening.

- Ask yourself, "Is there anything that I can do that will make a significant difference in the situation and how I'm feeling? And if so, am I willing to do it?" If you are struggling with your choices, reexamine what the other options were and why you made the decision you did. If you still feel that you made the correct decision and don't want or aren't willing to change your course of action, then you've done what you considered to be the right thing. Feeling guilty won't make it easier.

- **Be realistic in your expectations.** Remind yourself that your time, resources, and skills are limited. Understand that there may be a gap between what you wanted and the reality of what was available.

- **Refuse to judge yourself.** Guilt comes from your idea of what is right or wrong. This is usually learned from our parents and our friends. It's a perspective you use to judge yourself, and it may not be accurate.

- **Move on with your life.** Allow yourself the opportunity to enjoy the life you hoped for once the decisions were made and the changes implemented. What's the point of making any adjustments if you won't allow them to make a difference?

- **Remember that you are doing the best that you can!** You may not have handled everything perfectly, but you have tried to do what was right, perhaps under difficult circumstances. You would probably support and applaud others if they were in your shoes, so be as loving and accepting of your own actions.

CAREGIVER SURVIVAL TIP

Life is full of transitions—which are ever changing. Keep in mind that what is happening today will likely be different tomorrow, a month from now, or even a year from now. Don't hold so tightly to the past or how you wish things were that you lose the beauty of the moment today. Appreciate the opportunity to make a difference—no matter how small—for someone you love.

"There are four kinds of people in the world:
Those who have been caregivers;
Those who currently are caregivers;
Those who will be caregivers;
And those who will need caregivers."
—Rosalynn Carter, former First Lady

Resources

MEDICARE, MEDICAID, SOCIAL SECURITY, AND VETERAN BENEFITS

Administration on Aging, www.aoa.gov

Benefits Checkup, www.benefitscheckup.org

Eldercare Locator, www.eldercare.gov

Medicaid, www.medicaid.gov

Medicare, www.medicare.gov

Senior Veterans Service Alliance, www.veteransaidbenefit.org

Social Security Administration, www.ssa.gov

US Department of Veterans Affairs, www.va.gov

Veteran Aid, www.veteranaid.org

CAREGIVER SUPPORT

Care Flash, www.careflash.com

Caregiver Action Network, www.caregiveraction.org

Family Caregiver Alliance, www.caregiver.org

Help Guide, www.helpguide.org

National Alliance for Caregiving, www.caregiving.org

National Association of Professional Geriatric Care Managers, www.caremanager.org

LONG-TERM CARE

AARP, www.aarp.org

Administration on Aging, Long-Term Care, www.longtermcare .gov

Active-Insights, the Home of the Beneficiary Book, www.active -insights.com

Caring Connections, www.caringinfo.org

Do Your Own Will, www.doyourownwill.com

Elder Law Answers, www.elderlawanswers.com

Genworth, www.genworth.com

Law Depot, www.lawdepot.com

Medic Alert Foundation, www.medicalert.com

Mental Health, www.mentalhealth.gov

National Association of Cognitive-Behavioral Therapists, www .nacbt.org

Senior Discounts, www.seniordiscount.com

The National Long-Term Care Ombudsman Resource Center, www.ltcombudsman.org

Index